LABORATORY MANUAL
AND
WORKBOOK FOR

MICROBIOLOGY
IN
HEALTH
AND
DISEASE

Sixth Edition

ROBERT FUERST, B.S., M.A., Ph.D.

Professor of Biology, Head of the Microbiology Research Laboratory,
Texas Woman's University, Denton, Texas

1978

W. B. SAUNDERS COMPANY · Philadelphia · London · Toronto

W. B. Saunders Company: West Washington Square
Philadelphia, PA 19105

1 St. Anne's Road
Eastbourne, East Sussex BN21 3UN, England

1 Goldthorne Avenue
Toronto, Ontario M8Z 5T9, Canada

Laboratory Manual and Workbook for
MICROBIOLOGY IN HEALTH AND DISEASE   ISBN   0-7216-3943-7

Last digit is the print number: 9   8   7   6   5   4   3   2   1

PREFACE

This laboratory manual has been updated from the earlier edition and all errors have been carefully removed; my apologies to those users who may find new errors resulting from the revision. The fourteenth edition of *Frobisher and Fuerst's Microbiology in Health and Disease,* revised by Robert Fuerst, is the text from which this manual has been prepared. However, the effectiveness of the manual is not limited to users of any specific text. The organization of the laboratory manual proceeds from introductory material on the microscope, morphology and staining of microorganisms to disinfection and sterilization, sanitation, immunity, and pathogenic microorganisms. This is a common sequence in teaching microbiology in many schools. The section on pathogenic microorganisms has been presented from the viewpoint of methods of transmission rather than by using morphologic characteristics as the primary organizational pattern. In preparing this manual the author has relied on his own experience in teaching this material as well as on the seemingly successful fifth edition which predated this revision. For clarity, each laboratory exercise is divided into Key Steps and Important Points.

The author believes that laboratory work in microbiology can be taught without exposing the students to highly pathogenic microorganisms, but that all cultures of microorganisms should be handled with caution. It is his belief that beginning students in microbiology have not developed their aseptic technique sufficiently to warrant the hazard of having them handle virulent cultures. The author also feels that one of the primary outcomes of laboratory experience in microbiology is the realistic development of aseptic technique. Therefore, the instructors should insist on rigid adherence to principles and practice of asepsis in the laboratory. There should be good carryover of the techniques learned in the laboratory to clinical situations involving the health professions.

The author is grateful to many co-workers who have helped develop these laboratory exercises by their comments and suggestions, to the innumerable students who have made criticisms over a period of years, and to the instructors who have used the previous edition and forwarded suggestions and comments to the publisher. Special appreciation is due to the originator of this manual, Lucille Sommermeyer, who regrettably chose not to participate in the preparation of this and the last two editions.

The format of the allergy clinic scratch test has been provided through the courtesy of Dr. Ben Fisch, whose encouragement and personal friendship have been invaluable to the author.

Thanks are extended also to Miss Becky Russo, who conducted some of the experiments.

The author also acknowledges with sincere gratitude the outstanding work by the staff of the W. B. Saunders Company, who were always ready to help and cooperate, and without whose expert workmanship this laboratory manual would not have been possible.

ROBERT FUERST

NOTE TO INSTRUCTORS

This laboratory manual has been prepared to help you in your busy program. To use it best, you must be thoroughly familiar with each experiment. To utilize the time allotted for laboratory periods to its maximum advantage, it is recommended that all supplies and equipment should be available and ready for use before the laboratory period begins. In some situations assistants will prepare and check required materials. In other situations students may be assigned certain tasks of preparing equipment. Laboratory instruction in microbiology requires a great deal of expert planning and organization in order that the students may utilize the time provided for maximum learning. The author has found it highly profitable to prepare a schedule before beginning the course. This schedule includes the days when media should be prepared for use by the students, days when media should be inoculated with cultures, when transfers of stock cultures should be made, and so on. Such a schedule, if carefully thought through, reduces the possibility of forgetting vital materials.

This revision presents some new illustrations which may or may not meet your approval as far as techniques in the laboratory are concerned; no illustrations were deleted from the last edition. These illustrations were included here because the author has taught many students how to inoculate, pipette, streak plates, etc., by these methods. They were found to be helpful tools in learning to *avoid contamination.* If your methods are slightly different from those shown in the illustrations they are certainly not wrong. Perhaps the student can learn how to do things in more than one way, but most important *learn what not to do* in the laboratory or in the hospital situation. It is hoped that other new illustrations and tables added throughout the manual will be of help to students.

Exercise 40 (Staphylococci and Streptococci) and Exercise 41 (Growth of Anaerobes) are entirely new. The importance of anaerobic infections in the health field can hardly be overemphasized. You will find Exercise 41 easy to perform, and the results are very rewarding.

Although this laboratory manual is too long and detailed for some courses in microbiology, the exercises are written so that if omission is necessary the continuity will not be lost. For the short courses in microbiology, parts of experiments might be omitted or some of the following exercises might be completely deleted: Exercises 8, 10–12,

14, 15, 17–19, 26, 27, 30 and 31. Some of the work in Unit IV might be used as out-of-class assignments. The author believes that this manual is comprehensive enough to meet the needs of the most extensive course in microbiology given in schools of nursing and allied health sciences as well as in many colleges and universities.

NOTE TO STUDENTS

All laboratory manuals are only as good as the time, thought, and effort that is put into them by students. This laboratory manual has been arranged for your convenience. Space has been provided for recording results. All tables which could have been preconstructed have been prepared for you. Although it would be possible to complete this laboratory manual from available source materials, your knowledge of microbiology will grow into a useful, practical body of information only if you carry out each experiment as assigned, make your own observations, and record the results you observe. This entire laboratory manual has been prepared and selected from a wealth of available materials, and selection has been made of those materials which are essential to your practice in the health professions. The latest terminology has been applied throughout, and if it has changed since the last edition a footnote to this effect gives the former usage as well. Microbiology is a practical science, and the information learned in the course, and especially in the laboratory, will be important in the daily care of patients.

CONTENTS

Laboratory Exercise 7

Laboratory Exercise 8

Laboratory Exercise 9

Laboratory Exercise 10

Laboratory Exercise 11

Laboratory Exercise 12

Laboratory Exercise 13

Laboratory Exercise 14

Laboratory Exercise 15

Laboratory Exercise 16

UNIT II

PHYSICAL AND CHEMICAL AGENTS AS METHODS OF INHIBITING AND/OR KILLING BACTERIA

Laboratory Exercise 17

Laboratory Exercise 18

UNIT III

EXPERIMENTS SHOWING SOME SOURCES OF INFECTION, AND DEMONSTRATIONS OF IMMUNIZING AGENTS

UNIT IV

PATHOGENIC MICROORGANISMS

A. PATHOGENS TRANSMITTED FROM THE INTESTINAL AND/OR URINARY TRACT

B. PATHOGENS TRANSMITTED FROM THE RESPIRATORY TRACT

Unit 1

INTRODUCTION TO THE USE OF THE MICROSCOPE

MORPHOLOGY OF BACTERIA, MOLDS, YEASTS AND PROTOZOA

STERILE TECHNIQUES AND THE PREPARATION OF MEDIA

STAINING TECHNIQUES

OTHER TECHNIQUES IN THE STUDY OF MICROORGANISMS

OBJECTIVES: 1. To help the student understand the work and the functions of the microbiology laboratory.
2. To present certain basic guide lines for laboratory activity.

KEY STEPS	IMPORTANT POINTS
1. Protect your health and the health of others.	1.1. The reason you are taking this course and laboratory is first of all to learn to protect your health and the health of others against pathogenic microorganisms *as long as you shall live.* 1.2. Every microorganism you are using in the laboratory must be considered a potential pathogen; you will learn that many are indeed pathogenic. 1.3. You never eat, drink or smoke in the laboratory, nor do you bring any food or soft drinks into the laboratory.
2. Keep the laboratory as neat as possible at all times.	2.1. Because working space is limited and work in microbiology requires a certain amount of "elbow" room, you should bring only essential articles to the laboratory (laboratory manual, textbooks, pencils, pen). If possible, your overcoat should remain in the hall. 2.2. Ask your laboratory instructor for a proper place for your purse, satchel, books, and so forth. 2.3. A cluttered mess of test tubes, culture plates and slides not only is unsightly but also usually indicates that the worker is confused and disorganized. Therefore, you should discard materials you no longer need in the place designated by the instructor.
3. Protect your clothing.	3.1. Stains are used in microbiology and occasionally they are spilled accidentally. These will stain your clothes permanently. Therefore, you should wear a laboratory coat, smock or long plastic apron while you are in the laboratory. Lately, paper aprons (fireproof) have become available; they can even be washed and will wear long enough for one laboratory semester.

4. Wash your hands and the laboratory desk with a 2% Lysol or Cresol solution, or at least with soap and water, at the beginning and the end of each laboratory period. For some students with sensitive skin, the use of a more expensive, but milder, disinfectant may be recommended for hand washing.

4.1. This removes dust, prevents unnecessary contamination and helps keep the laboratory tidy.

4.2. pHisoDerm, a milder disinfectant, has replaced pHisoHex, often used for washing hands.

5. At the end of each laboratory period check and arrange neatly all equipment assigned to you.

5.1. In order to assure that you will have your allocated equipment, it is important to replace missing and broken materials at the end of each laboratory period.

6. Moisten the labels and pencils with water from the tap, kept in some convenient container on the working table—but *never* with your tongue.

6.1. Placing any articles, or even your fingers, in your mouth is a method of transfer of microorganisms.

6.2. Your laboratory instructor can help you to break the bad and dangerous habit of putting your pencil into your mouth by saying "fomite" every time you do it.

7. Keep your hands away from the region of your face and head during a laboratory period.

7.1. Your hands may be soiled, stained or contaminated.

8. Keep your hair under control.

8.1. Long, uncontrolled hair and non-fireproof clothing are fire hazards in the laboratory where Bunsen burners will be lit. When you smell burning hair, it usually is in contact with or too close to the open flame.

9. Avoid setting things on fire.

9.1. Fires will occur in every microbiology laboratory. It's usually cotton that burns. Stay cool; don't blow at the fire. Putting your hand over the cotton will help, or step on it— smother the fire.

9.2. Most important, the laboratory instructor will demonstrate use of the fire extinguisher in your laboratory to you.

10. Report all accidents to the instructor. (This includes minor cuts, abrasions, pricks and burns, as well as major injuries.)

10.1. Minor injuries can be treated adequately with first-aid measures. If these injuries are untreated, they may result in much more serious conditions.

10.2. Burns are best treated with ice and cold water, applied immediately. Sodium bicarbonate (baking soda) liberally applied to the burn will reduce the pain.

KEY STEPS	IMPORTANT POINTS
	10.3. More serious injuries should be referred immediately to the medical center.
11. Leave all teaching materials in the laboratory.	11.1. There is no excuse for storing cultures and specimens in your room. 11.2. Cultures, specimens and illustrative material need to be shared with other students in the class.
12. Discard all solid waste material in containers provided for this purpose.	12.1. Materials like paper, cotton and media will clog the plumbing if these substances are put in the sink.
13. Check with your instructor about disposal of unused sterile materials and the return of special equipment.	13.1. These materials may be needed for other students.
14. Before leaving the laboratory, wash your hands thoroughly with 2% Lysol solution, Cresol, pHisoDerm, other mild disinfectants, or at least soap and running water.	14.1. Hands may be a method of transferring microorganisms from the laboratory to your nose and mouth and to others.

OBJECTIVES: 1. To help the student understand the need for preparations for each laboratory period.
2. To help the student develop scientific methods of approach to laboratory problems.

KEY STEPS	IMPORTANT POINTS
1. Carefully read the directions of each experiment before beginning your work.	1.1. This helps you to know what you are going to do. 1.2. In addition to knowing the steps of an experiment you should also understand its purpose. 1.3. If you do not understand completely, ask questions. "The wise man knows what he does not know."
2. Before doing an experiment, state *in writing* what you expect to learn from this experience in the laboratory.	2.1. Writing your expected learnings helps to clarify the purpose of the experiment and focus your attention on this learning experience.
3. If the experiment fails to yield the expected results, explain why.	3.1. Recognition of why an experiment fails may be as important to your learning as the success of an experiment.
4. Develop good habits of technique as demonstrated for you and as described in the laboratory experiments.	4.1. Microbiologic laboratory technique is very important to you because of its direct relation to many technical methods used in the health fields. 4.2. Sometimes a student accidentally drops some glassware containing bacteria. Immediately pour 2% Lysol solution over the entire area splattered with glass and liquid. After some time clean it up with a mop and broom. (Take care not to cut yourself.) Wash your hands with 2% Lysol. This is to protect your health and that of others. 4.3. If cultures are accidentally spilled, report this to the instructor immediately and state if the material has been adequately disinfected. However, this type of accident should be avoided at all times.
5. Report results of laboratory experiments on sheets provided in this manual. Use clear, concise statements. Use charts and drawings as frequently as possible.	5.1. Accurate reporting is a function of all individuals working in areas of science. Students should develop good habits of reporting as early in the educational program as possible. 5.2. Charts and drawings may tell the story better than any description.

KEY STEPS	IMPORTANT POINTS
6. Drawings should be clear, in good proportions and done with a hard pencil.	6.1. You are not expected to be an artist. Clear, diagrammatic drawings are all that are required. 6.2. Do not use shading because, in drawings of microscopic organisms, shading obscures the essentials. 6.3. You may color your drawings to represent various stains, if you wish. If you use colors, make them as true to the color of the stain as possible. 6.4. Draw only what you can see under the microscope; copying from a book will not help you to perfect your laboratory technique. 6.5. It is usually best to make your final drawing in the laboratory directly from what you see and not to rely on memory or sketches on scraps of paper made for later transfer.
7. Answer all questions at the end of each experiment.	7.1. The answers to the questions may be found in the results of the experiments, in your textbook, or in reference books, or they may force you to think in terms of the material you have studied. The latter is often resented by some students, but really helps in the learning process.
8. Ask for help from the instructor if needed during the laboratory period.	8.1. The instructor is available to help students but may not always recognize that you are having difficulty. 8.2. If you do not understand the relationship between lectures and laboratory, ask the instructor to help you. 8.3. If you do not understand the relationship between this course and your major field of studies, ask questions. One of the most important purposes of a course in microbiology is to help you to be a better and more intelligent person, and most of all to recognize the effects of microorganisms on the health and disease of people.

Laboratory Exercise 1

TOPIC: THE USE AND CARE OF THE MICROSCOPE

OBJECTIVES:
1. To introduce the student to the applications of the microscope as a laboratory tool.
2. To demonstrate the correct ways of using a microscope.
3. To help the student to understand the precautions that must be taken to protect the microscope from damage.

KEY STEPS	IMPORTANT POINTS
A. _Care of the Microscope:_ 1. Learn the essential points about the use of a microscope.	1.1. In order to finish the assigned exercises, it is desirable that students learn how to focus on an object with a microscope.
2. Keep the body of the microscope in a perpendicular position.	2.1. Students who are beginning to use a microscope may have serious accidents with spilling of moist materials on a microscope if they tilt the body tube. 2.2. The body tube of a microscope is **never** tilted when using the oil immersion objectives. 2.3. Experienced workers who must use the microscope for many hours may tilt the body tube when examining **dry** preparations with the high dry objective.
3. If your microscope is not functioning properly, report it to your instructor.	3.1. Your instructor will be able to determine if major or minor adjustments need to be made.
4. Keep the stage clean and dry.	4.1. Liquids or dirt on the stage may be transferred to the lenses. This might result in serious damage to the microscope.
5. Clean lenses with lens paper only.	5.1. Lens paper is a very fine paper which will not scratch or damage sensitive lenses. 5.2. If dry lens paper is not sufficient to clean the lenses, the lens paper may be moistened with a **small amount** of xylene (also called xylol) to facilitate cleaning. 5.3. If any lens remains foggy after your best efforts of cleaning, report it to the instructor, who will assist you.

KEY STEPS	IMPORTANT POINTS
	5.4. If there is dirt on the ocular (determined by rotating the ocular slowly: if the dirt rotates with the ocular you have determined the source), clean the upper surface with lens paper. If you cannot remove the dirt by cleaning the upper surface, notify the instructor. 5.5. Until you are proficient in the use of a microscope, you should not remove any lenses from it without permission of the instructor.
6. Use special immersion oil (preferably Crown, Cargill's or Shillaber's oil) with the oil immersion lens.	6.1. The oil immersion lens on the longest objective gives the highest magnification. 6.2. The high magnification of the oil immersion objective is made possible because the oil used has almost the same power of refraction as the glass of the lens. 6.3. Immersion oil is the only liquid which touches the glass of the oil immersion lens. 6.4. The oil immersion lens is the most expensive one on your microscope. Give it the best care possible.
7. Always carry the microscope with two hands.	7.1. Microscopes should be transported from place to place with utmost care in an upright position. 7.2. When carrying a microscope outside its case, one hand should support the base and one hand should grasp the carrying arm.
8. Place the microscope on the desk gently.	8.1. While the microscope appears to be a sturdy instrument, it is a delicate, precise piece of equipment which has been assembled with extreme care. 8.2. Sudden jarring can ruin its precision alignment and can result in a poorly functioning microscope.
9. When you leave a microscope, clean all lenses that you have used.	9.1. Dust may accumulate on lenses and result in a film which is difficult to remove. This film does not form if lenses are cleaned frequently.
10. When you leave a microscope, place the low power objective in position over the opening in the stage.	10.1. On all new microscopes the body tube has a stop for the low power objective. This stop prevents the tip of the objective from any contact with the lens of the substage condenser. 10.2. The high dry and oil immersion objectives do not have a stop and may be damaged by accidental contact with the substage condenser.

KEY STEPS	IMPORTANT POINTS
11. When you finish using the microscope, return it to its case or cover it with a plastic protector.	11.1. Covering a microscope protects it from unnecessary dust and dirt.
B. *Focusing a Microscope:* 1. Move the microscope so that it is directly in front of you on the laboratory table.	1.1. The back of the base should be at the edge of the table. 1.2. The two arms of the base should be pointing away from you at right angles to the edge of the table. 1.3. Note that some microscopes are now so constructed that exactly the reverse of 1.1 and 1.2 is true ***for their use.***
2. Use light from a microscope lamp, unless your microscope has built-in illumination.	2.1. Indirect sunlight reflected from the clouds used to be the most acceptable source of light for microscope work, but its use has been discontinued, since electric light results in a more stable and controllable illumination. 2.2. The source of light is either reflected through a mirror, up the microscope toward the eye(s) of the observer or, in more ***modern*** instruments, the light source is mounted directly underneath the objective and the upward light beam can be controlled by means of a transformer.
3. Use the concave side of the mirror for artificial light, unless your microscope has built-in substage illumination.	3.1. The concave mirror reflects the greatest number of light rays through the condenser. 3.2. The mirror should be adjusted until it is obvious that a large concentration of light rays are passing through the substage condenser. 3.3. The light is optimum when a clear, uniform circle of light is visible when you are looking through the ocular. 3.4. The condenser and diaphragm aid in adjusting the intensity of the available light. 3.5. Experience in focusing will help you in judging the optimum light requirements for microscopic work.
4. Adjust the condenser so that it is flush with the stage.	4.1. When the condenser is in this position, the maximum amount of light is focused through the microscope.
5. Using clips or the mechanical stage will hold the slide to be studied on the stage so that the center of the material on the slide is directly over the lens of the condenser.	5.1. By placing the slide in this position, you will be most likely to have the material you want to study in the correct position for focusing.

KEY STEPS	IMPORTANT POINTS
6. While you observe the distance between the tip of the objective and the slide, *look at the side of the microscope* and carefully lower the objective toward the slide. *Do not allow the tip of any objective to touch the slide.*	6.1. The lenses of objectives may be badly scratched if they contact a glass slide. 6.2. While this precaution is not as essential when using the low power objective as when using either of the other two objectives, it is important to develop habits so that you will always observe the distance between the objective and the slide. After you have developed these habits, you will *never* look in the ocular while the objective is moving toward the slide.
7. Focus first with the low power objective whenever you are uncertain of the location of the microscopic material on the glass slide.	7.1. The low power objective gives you the lowest magnification (usually $\times$ 100). 7.2. It is usually easier to find the object with the low power objective than the higher magnifications. 7.3. When using the low power objective, the object comes into focus when the lens of the objective is about 16 mm from the slide.
8. If your microscope has only one ocular (eyepiece) look through the ocular with one eye while keeping both eyes open.	8.1. Closing one eye while working with a microscope may result in eyestrain. 8.2. It is easiest for the beginning student to learn to keep both eyes open if you practice tilting your head to the side of the eye you are using to look through the ocular. 8.3. Note that all research microscopes have two oculars to eliminate eyestrain. This also permits adjusting the setting of the second ocular to the visual needs of the person using the microscope, after the first ocular has been focused.
9. While looking through the ocular, move the objective *slowly away* (up) from the slide by turning the coarse adjustment knob (in most microscopes) *counterclockwise.*	9.1. If you turn the coarse adjustment knob too rapidly, you will be likely to pass the focus of the object without seeing it. 9.2. If you pass the point where the object comes into focus, you will have to lower the objective by raising your head and observing from the side of the microscope, as described in Step 6.
10. When the object is focused as well as possible with the coarse adjustment knob, adjust and sharpen the focus further with the fine adjustment knob.	10.1. By turning the fine adjustment knob with both clockwise and counterclockwise movements, you are moving the objective down and up. 10.2. This movement with the fine adjustment knob is not visible with the naked eye but must be remembered when the objective is close to the slide.

KEY STEPS	**IMPORTANT POINTS**

10.3. If the fine adjustment knob will not move in one direction or seems to be stuck, ask the instructor to help you with this adjustment until you learn to do it yourself.

11. After you have focused on the object clearly with the low power objective, turn the high power objective into position by moving it into place over the slide.

11.1. The modern microscope is adjusted so that objects in view with one power of magnification are in focus with a different magnification. Unfortunately, with extensive use of the microscope, this convenient feature may not persist.

11.2. You may need to sharpen the focus with the fine adjustment knob.

11.3. You will need to remember that changing from a low magnification to a high magnification decreases the diameter of the material that you will see. Therefore, it is important that the particular material that you want to see with a higher magnification is in the center of the field as you see it with a lower magnification.

11.4. The usual magnification of the microscope with the high dry power objective in place, and using the $\times$ 10 eyepiece, is $\times$ 430 to $\times$ 460.

12. Learn to use the low power and high power objectives well, before you proceed to learn the use of the oil immersion lens.

12.1. If you have not had extensive experience with a microscope before, it is wise to learn the simpler procedures of focusing with the 16 mm and 4 mm objectives well, prior to learning the more complex oil immersion techniques. You will find your material on the slides much more quickly and with less danger of breakage after you have done so.

13. To use the oil immersion lens for focusing, raise the objective from the slide, place a drop of immersion oil on the slide, swing the oil immersion objective into place and by turning the coarse objective knob, lower the tip of this objective into the drop of oil.

13.1. The oil immersion objective has the shortest focal distance, i.e., about 1.8 mm from the object.

13.2. You should *always* observe the distance between the tip of the oil immersion objective and the slide, by looking at it from the side of the microscope, when you are moving the objective downward.

13.3. The tip of the objective should be well immersed in the *oil* but *should not touch the slide.*

KEY STEPS	**IMPORTANT POINTS**
14. While looking into the ocular, focus away from the slide *slowly* by turning the *fine* adjustment knob.	14.1. Because the focal distance is close to the slide, you will miss the object completely if you use the coarse adjustment knob for focusing or if you turn the fine adjustment knob too rapidly. 14.2. If you turn the fine adjustment knob in a counterclockwise direction, this usually moves the objective away from the slide. Check with your instructor about this before you start. 14.3. If you miss the object by going beyond the focal distance and the objective is above the drop of oil, you must lower the objective again into the oil as explained in Steps 12 and 13. 14.4. The magnification of the microscope when you are using the oil immersion objective is approximately $\times$ 960 to $\times$ 1,000.
15. Observe your slides with careful thought for detail.	15.1. The care you use in making observations will be evident in your drawings. 15.2. After making careful observations, draw what you have seen. 15.3. Drawings of microscopic objects should be large enough to show observed details.
16. After you have completed your observations with the oil immersion lens, use the coarse adjustment knob to raise the objective from the slide, remove the slide from the stage and wipe the excess oil from the lens of the objective with dry lens paper. Then use a very small amount of xylene on the lens paper to remove any traces of oil on the microscope and objective and again wipe dry.	16.1. If nonhardening oil (Crown, Cargill's or Shillaber's oil) is used, cleaning with dry lens paper may be sufficient.
17. Put your microscope away clean and in good condition.	17.1. See Steps 9, 10 and 11, pages 10 and 11.
18. There is actually no need for using the high or low power objectives if you know that the material to be observed requires the use of the oil immersion lens *provided you have obtained sufficient skill* in the use of the microscope.	18.1. If you have sufficient skill in the use of the microscope, especially using oil immersion, you may omit Key Steps 7 to 11 and proceed immediately but carefully to Step 13. Only your instructor can advise you if you have *mastered* the use of your microscope.

C. *Some Magnifications Possible with the Compound Microscope:*

Name	Objective Focal Length	Magnification	Eyepiece Magnification	Total Magnification
Low power	16 mm	× 10	× 10	× 100
	16 mm	× 10	× 12	× 120
High dry	4 mm	× 44	× 10	× 440
	4 mm	× 44	× 15	× 660
Oil immersion	1.8 mm	× 95	× 8	× 760
	1.8 mm	× 95	× 10	× 950

Laboratory Exercise 2

TOPIC: IDENTIFICATION OF THE PARTS OF THE MICROSCOPE

OBJECTIVE: 1. To help the student to know the names of the parts of the microscope.

DIRECTIONS: Label all parts of the diagrammatic drawing of the microscope. You may study first the information given at the end of this exercise, but do not just copy the words. This will not help you to learn.

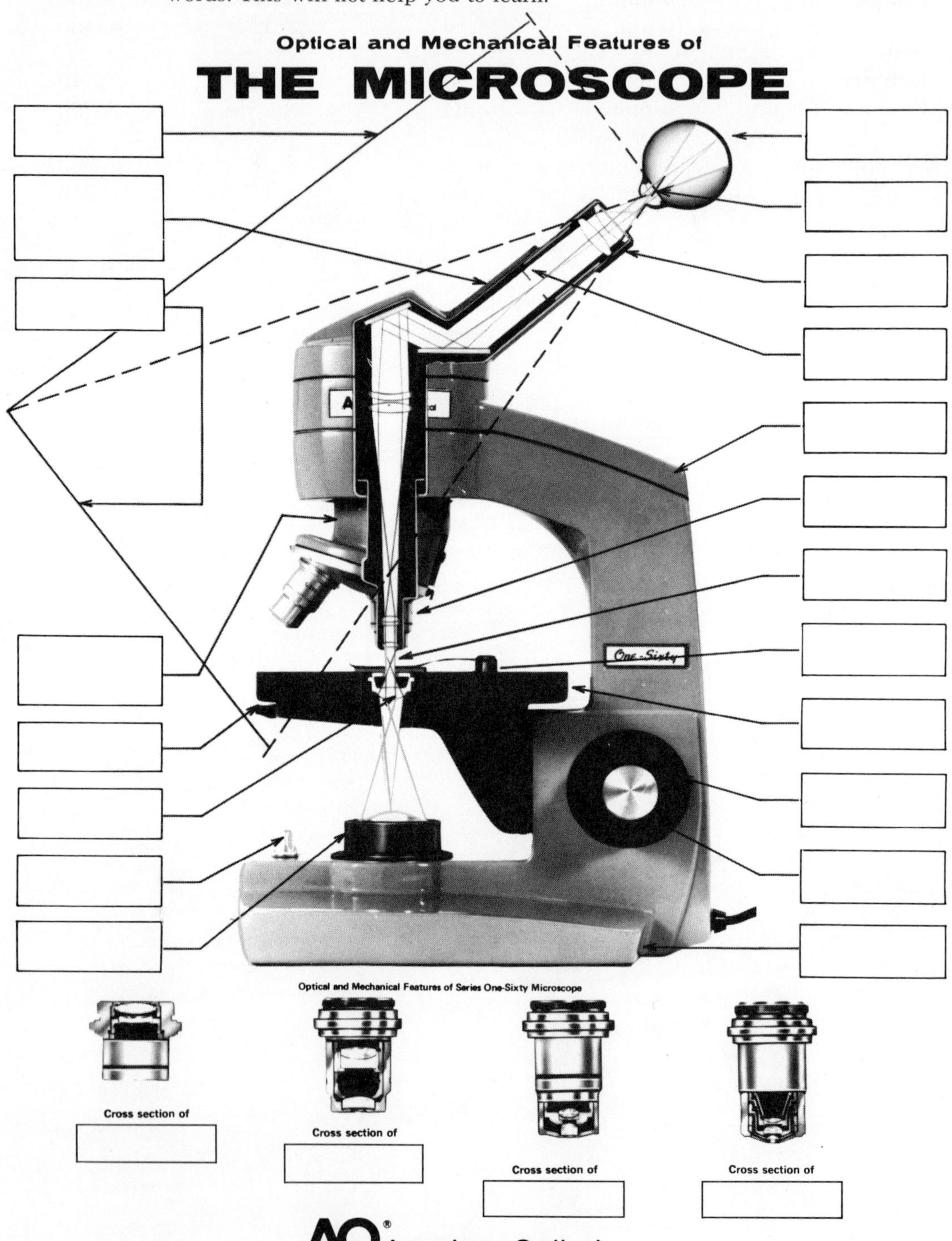

AO® American Optical
SCIENTIFIC INSTRUMENT DIVISION
BUFFALO, NY 14215

® Reg. TM American Optical Corporation
Please write for authorization to use in textbooks and laboratory manuals.

TOPIC: FUNCTIONS OF PARTS OF THE MICROSCOPE

OBJECTIVES: 1. To help the student to understand the functions of the parts of the microscope.
2. To help the student to understand the magnification that is possible with the microscope.

Questions:

1. State briefly the functions of each of the following parts:

Eyepiece (ocular) ____

Body tube ____

____

Revolving nose piece ____

Objectives ____

Stage ____

Stage clip ____

Mechanical stage ____

A mechanical stage with graduated scales ____

____

In-stage or substage condenser ____

____

Disc aperture diaphragm ____

Mirror ____

Inclination joint (in older microscopes) ____

Base ____

Arm ____

Coarse adjustment knob ____

____

Fine adjustment knob ____

____

2. Give a proper magnification for each of the following objective settings, or parts, on your microscope:

Eyepiece (ocular) ____

Low power objective ____

High dry power objective ____

Oil immersion objective ____

The magnification of the microscope with the $\times 10$ eyepiece and the low power

objective in place is ____

____

The magnification of the microscope with the $\times 15$ eyepiece and the high dry power

objective in place is ____

____

The magnification of the microscope with the $\times 10$ eyepiece and the oil immersion

objective in place is ____

____

TOPIC: THE PARTS AND THE USE OF THE MICROSCOPE

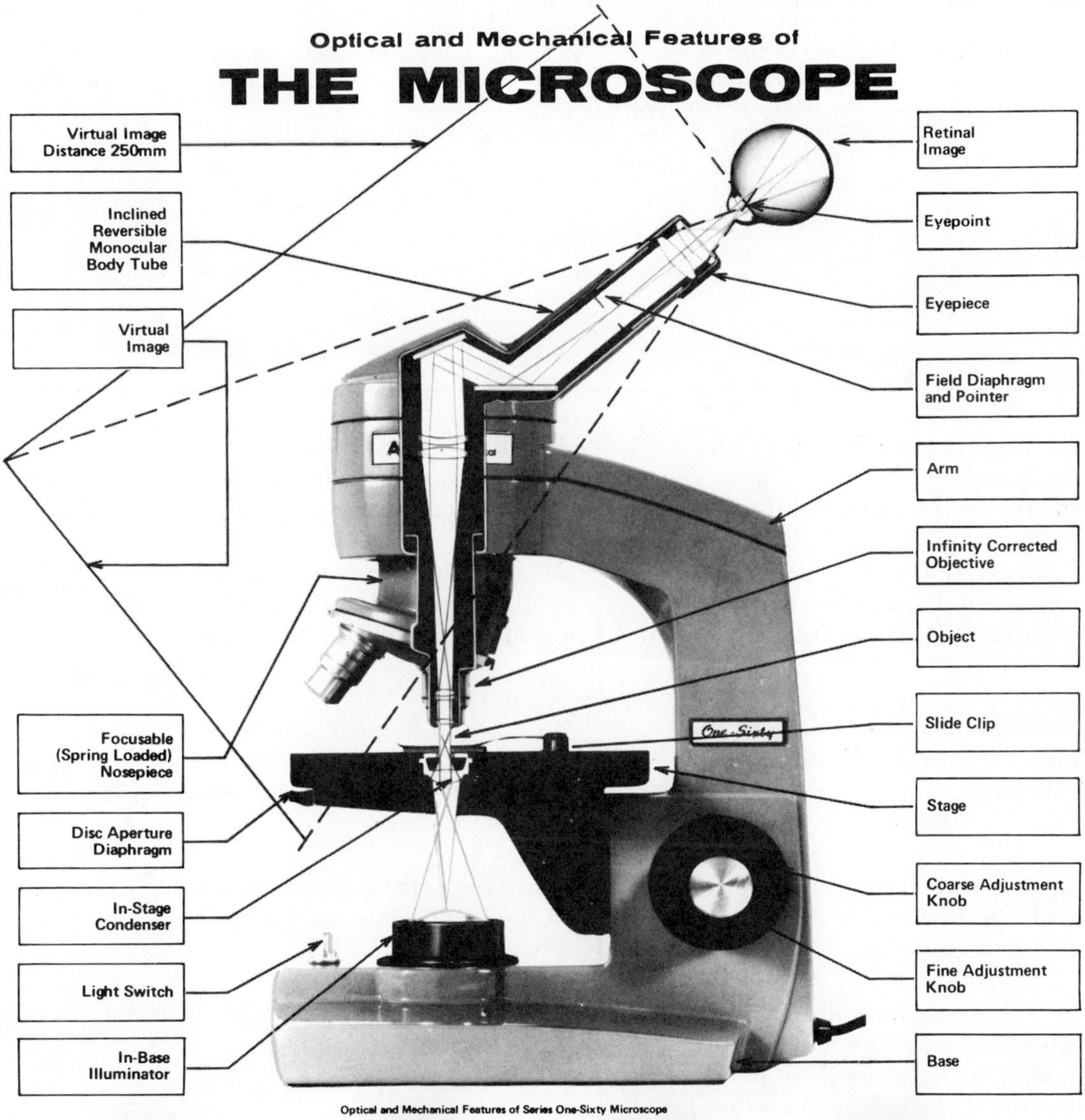

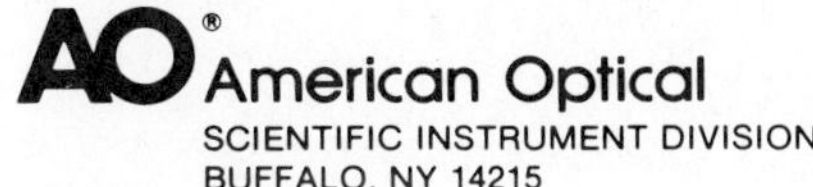

American Optical

SCIENTIFIC INSTRUMENT DIVISION
BUFFALO, NY 14215

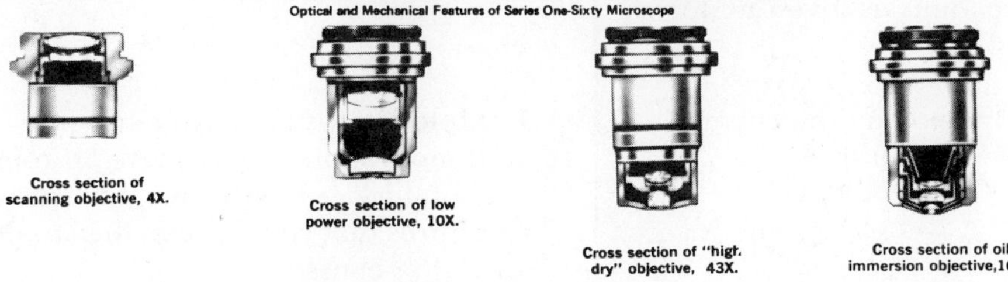

® Reg. TM American Optical Corporation
Please write for authorization to use in textbooks and laboratory manuals.

Laboratory Exercise 3

TOPIC: MOLDS

OBJECTIVE: 1. To examine briefly the structure of molds.

EQUIPMENT: 1. Pure culture of molds (if possible, have one culture of septate mold, and one of nonseptate mold; also, have one specimen which shows sporangia and one which shows conidia).
2. Moldy bread, cheese, fruits (oranges) and other sources of mold.
3. Hollow-ground slides.
4. Coverslips.

Procedure:

KEY STEPS	IMPORTANT POINTS
1. Take a clean, hollow-ground slide and a clean coverslip to your instructor for a sample of mold.	1.1. Because mold spores are easily disseminated, it is advisable that molds should be handled only by experienced people.
2. As soon as you receive your sample of mold in the hollow-ground slide, cover it with a clean coverslip.	2.1. Covering your sample will keep it in the well of the hollow-ground slide until you can examine it with the microscope.
3. Examine your sample of mold under low and high power magnification.	3.1. Try to identify mycelia, hyphae, sporangia (if present) and conidia (if present). 3.2. Look for cross walls (septa) in the mycelia.
4. Examine a sample of moldy food with the low power magnification of the microscope.	4.1. You will be able to see the formations of the mold plant on food.
5. Take a clean, hollow-ground slide and a clean coverslip to the instructor for a small bit of food. Follow directions as given under Steps 2 and 3.	5.1. See Steps 1.1., 2.1., 3.1., and 3.2.
6. Without removing the coverslips, return the slides to the instructor.	6.1. Mold spores are easily airborne. 6.2. If mold spores are scattered throughout the laboratory, you will have them growing in the cultures that you make in the laboratory later in the course.

Record of Results:

1. Make drawings of a portion of each sample as seen under both low and high power magnification. Record in spaces provided.
   a. Show differences in structure in those samples.
   b. Watch for details and include these in your drawings.
   c. Always check and record your magnification as soon as you have focused in on the material.

Questions:

1. A mold conidium is ____

   ____

2. A mycelium is ____

   ____

3. Two diseases of man which may be caused by mold or moldlike organisms are

   ____

   and ____

4. List the reasons why precautions must be taken to keep mold cultures under control in the laboratory.

5. List the precautions which can be taken by the housewife to reduce the loss of food from mold contamination.

6. From observations of the way molds grow, state why it is often so difficult to destroy them when they are infecting living tissue.

7. State the advantages to man that have been discovered by studying the products of molds.

Drawings of Molds

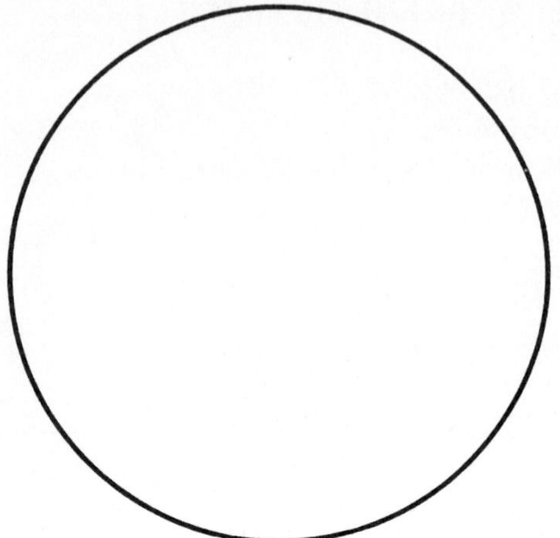

Figure 3–1. Object _______________

Magnification ×_______

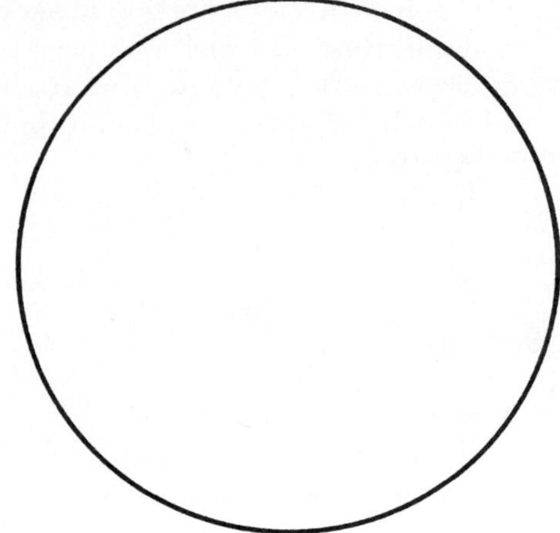

Figure 3–2. Object_______________

Magnification ×_______

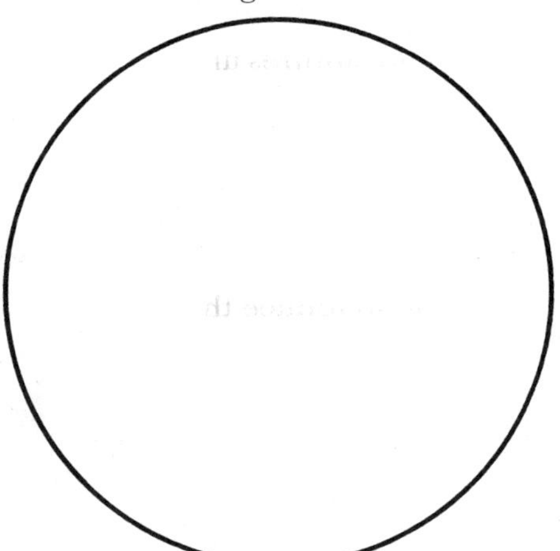

Figure 3–3. Object _______________

Magnification ×_______

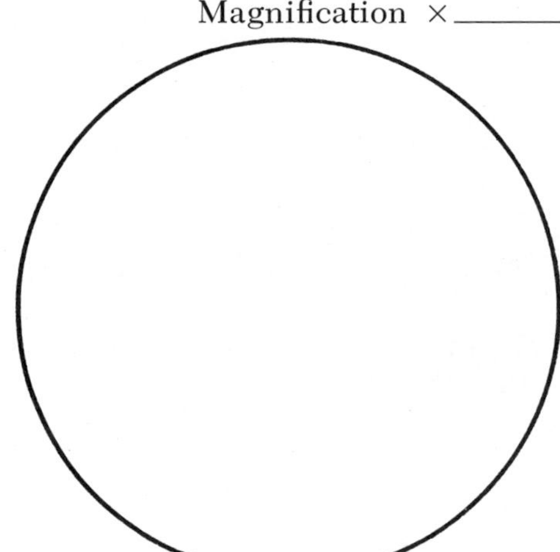

Figure 3–4. Object _______________

Magnification ×_______

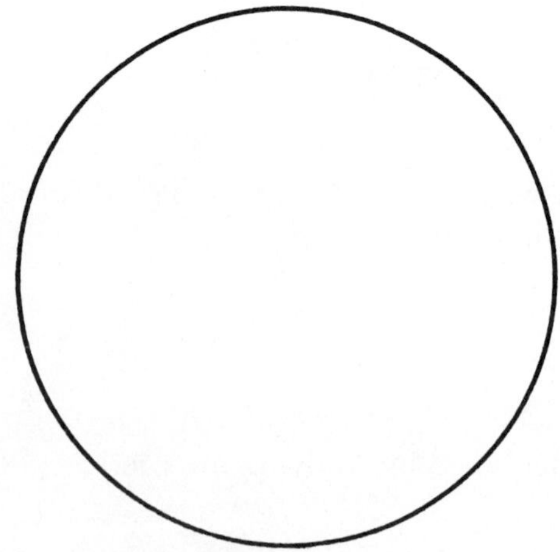

Figure 3–5. Object _______________

Magnification ×_______

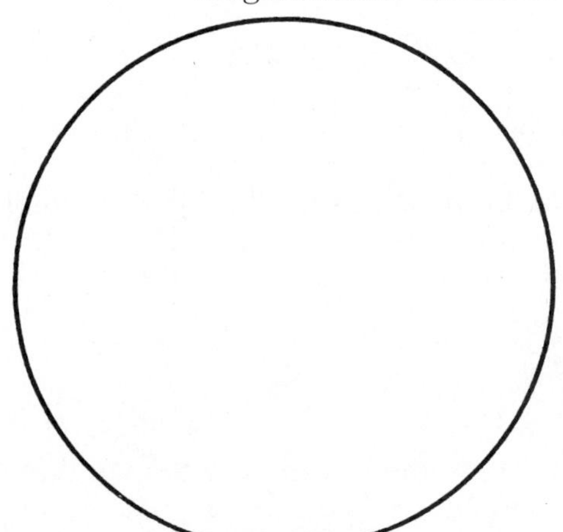

Figure 3–6. Object _______________

Magnification ×_______

Laboratory Exercise 4

TOPIC: YEASTS IN A HANGING DROP

OBJECTIVE: 1. To help the student to understand the structure and reproduction of yeasts.

EQUIPMENT: 1. Sucrose broth culture of *Saccharomyces cerevisiae* (bakers' yeast).
2. 24 hr culture of yeast in starch solution.
3. Clean hollow-ground glass slides.
4. Clean coverslips.
5. 5% Lysol, 5% phenol solution or 5% saponated solution of cresol in a large beaker.
6. Gram's iodine solution, if step 12.2. will be done as an exercise.

Procedure:

Note that illustrations of the laboratory techniques you will use in this experiment and many others are shown at the end of this exercise.

KEY STEPS	IMPORTANT POINTS
1. Thoroughly clean the hollow-ground slide and the coverslip.	1.1. Dust and fingerprints are magnified when the object is enlarged by looking in a microscope.
2. Obtain a broth culture of the yeast *Saccharomyces cerevisiae* from your instructor.	2.1. This culture has been prepared by growing yeast in a solution of sucrose and beef broth. 2.2. *Saccharomyces cerevisiae* is commonly known as bakers' yeast.
3. Flame your inoculating loop and allow it to cool.	3.1. In order to flame an inoculating loop, hold the handle of the loop near the Bunsen burner so that the wire loop becomes red hot for its entire length; flame from the handle toward the end of the wire. This destroys all microorganisms which might be on the loop. Don't rush when you reach the loop. Be certain it too is well flamed. 3.2. After getting the wire red hot, remove it from the flame and let it cool by holding it in the air a short time. ***Do not lay it down.*** Hold the needle like a pencil, as is usually done by most people.
4. Remove the cotton plug (or the cap) from the mouth of the tube.	4.1. The cotton plug (or the cap) can be removed best by grasping the outer portion of the plug with the little finger and edge of the palm of the same hand in which the loop needle is held. Some people prefer to hold the plug between the first and second fingers or between the third and fourth fingers. 4.2. ***Do not palm the cotton plug*** (or the cap), since this contaminates every surface where the hand touches it.

KEY STEPS	IMPORTANT POINTS
	4.3. The inner portion of the cotton plug (or the cap) should point away from your hand and body. 4.4. It is very important that you should *avoid touching the inside of the cotton plug (or the cap) (the part that goes back into the tube) with anything.*
5. Insert the sterile inoculating loop into the culture tube and obtain a loopful of the liquid.	5.1. This is the beginning of your practice with sterile technique. 5.2. You are trying to transfer living microorganisms from the culture tube to the slide without contaminating the culture in the tube and without transferring the organism to any place other than the slide.
6. Replace the cotton plug in the mouth of the culture tube, or the cap on the tube opening.	6.1. The cotton plug filters air and prevents other microorganisms from entering the tube. If a cap is used, it should not be too tight on the tube and it should extend far enough down on the outside (3.8 cm) so it could not possibly fall off.
7. Place the drop of the culture (see Step 5) on the center of the clean coverslip lying on a clean paper or towel.	7.1. This drop must be placed in the center so that it is suspended as a drop when inverted.
8. Flame the inoculating loop.	8.1. See Steps 3.1 and 3.2. 8.2. The inoculating loop must be flamed at this point to avoid transferring microorganisms to your desk. To avoid splatter, again flame from the handle toward the loop. Do this slowly. (Why?)
9. Rim the edge of the depression in the hollow-ground slide with water or with a *very* thin film of water-soluble lubricant. Do not allow any water or lubricant to get into the depression of the slide. Place the slide on a paper or towel on the table.	9.1. This thin film of water or Vaseline will permit the coverslip to adhere more securely to the slide. 9.2. Water or lubricant in the depression will prevent visibility of the material on the coverslip.
10. Pick up the coverslip (from Step 7) with your thumb and forefinger and invert your hand, holding the coverslip gently so that the hanging drop of the culture is over the center of the depression on the slide.	10.1. By turning the coverslip over quickly, and following with Step 11, it will remain adhered to the slip, and the drop of culture (hanging drop) will become suspended in the depression of the hollow-ground slide. 10.2. The drop of the culture should hang suspended in the space of the depression of the hollow-ground slide.

KEY STEPS	**IMPORTANT POINTS**
11. *Gently* press the coverslip to the hollow-ground slide.	11.1. This slight pressure will adhere the coverslip to the slide. 11.2. If this simple procedure should give you difficulties, you can always put a drop of the yeast culture on a clean slide, add a drop of dilute iodine solution, put the coverslip over the yeast and examine the slide under the microscope.
12. Examine the hanging drop with low and high power magnification.	12.1. The yeast cells will show certain characteristics which are different from molds and, as you will see later, also bacteria. 12.2. The yeast cultures will be actively reproducing. Notice the way in which they reproduce.
13. Look at the culture of yeast in starch solution and compare with the culture made in sucrose broth.	13.1. There are differences in what this micro-organism does in each of these solutions.
14. Immerse the slide, with the coverslip still attached, in a beaker containing 5% Lysol, a 5% solution of phenol or a 5% solution of saponated cresol.	14.1. Yeast cells can be destroyed by these disinfectants. 14.2. This procedure should be followed whenever you discard a hanging drop slide of living organisms.

Record of Results:

1. Draw yeast cells under low and high dry power in spaces provided.
2. Record the changes which have occurred in the yeast cultures.

Questions:

1. Yeasts have the ability to decompose carbohydrates (sugars) into ___________

   and _______________. This process is known as _____________________.

2. Two important uses for yeast cells are ___________________________ and

   ____.

3. Yeasts reproduce by _____________________________________

4. Two diseases of man caused by yeastlike organisms are _________________

   _________________ and _________________________________.

DRAWINGS OF YEASTS

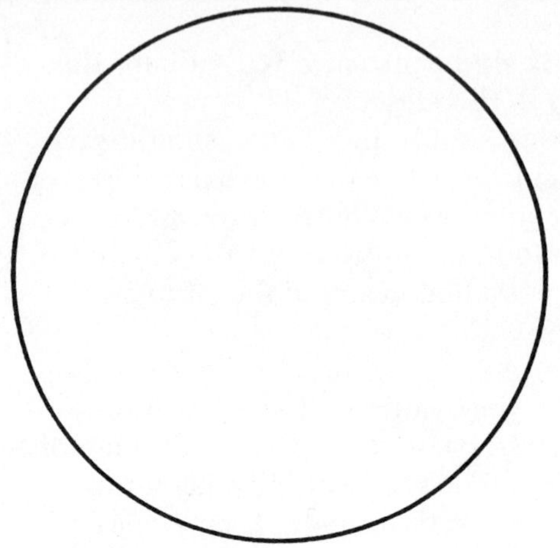

Figure 4–1. Object________________

Magnification ×________

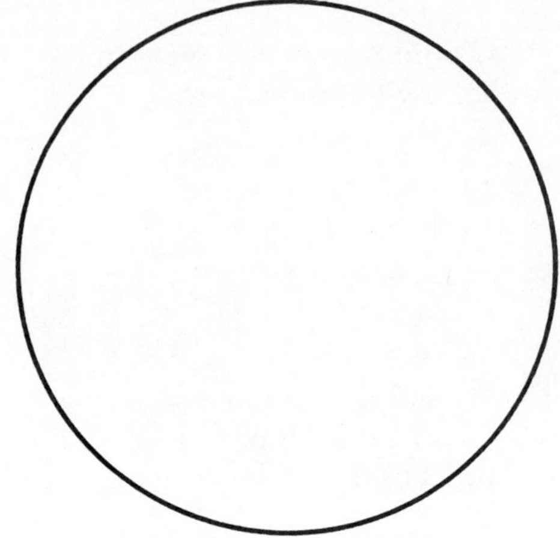

Figure 4–2. Object________________

Magnification ×________

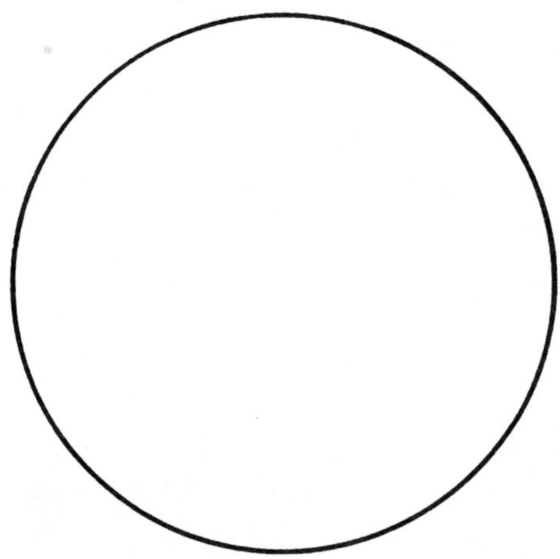

Figure 4–3. Object________________

Magnification ×________

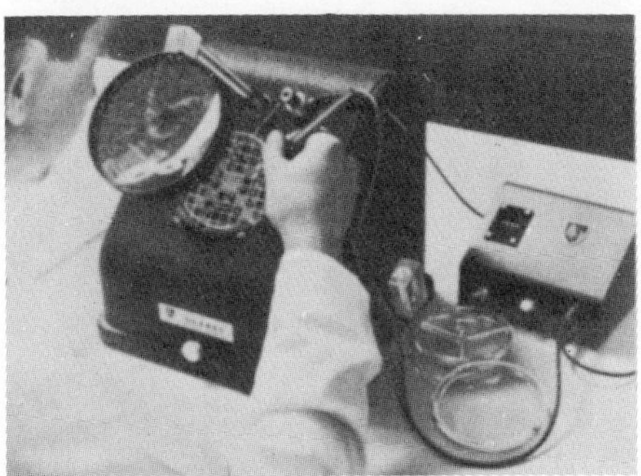

1. A QUEBEC Colony Counter. The open Petri plate is placed over the light, below the magnifier glass. The hand counter is used to record the number of bacterial colonies per plate.

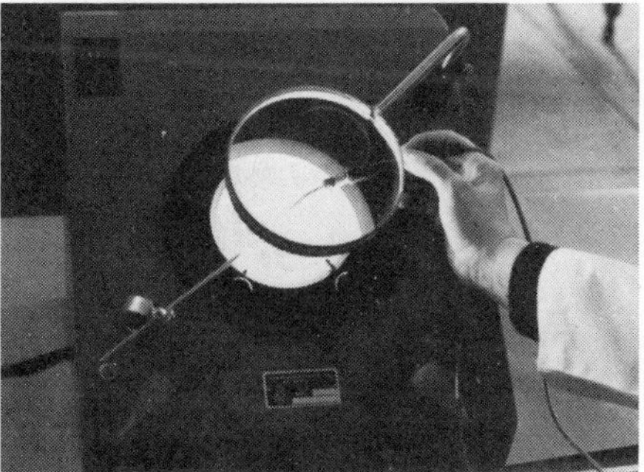

2. An improved type of bacterial colony counter. Contact is made between the machine and the agar in the plate through a rod on the left. The probe in the right hand is used to touch the colonies and the electric contact activates the digital counter.

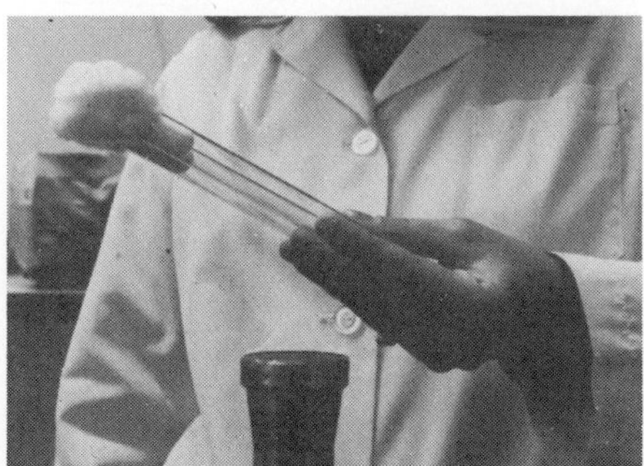

3. This figure shows how test tubes are held to inoculate microorganisms from one tube into another one. The tubes are held like an extension of the fingers; the thumb is on top.

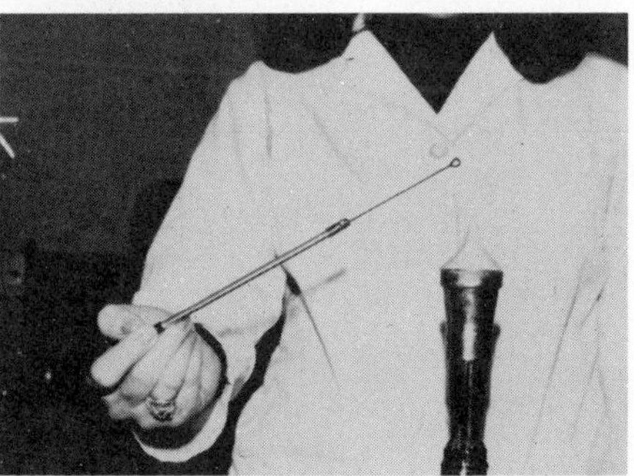

4. The loop needle is held like a pencil in the right hand, for right handed people.

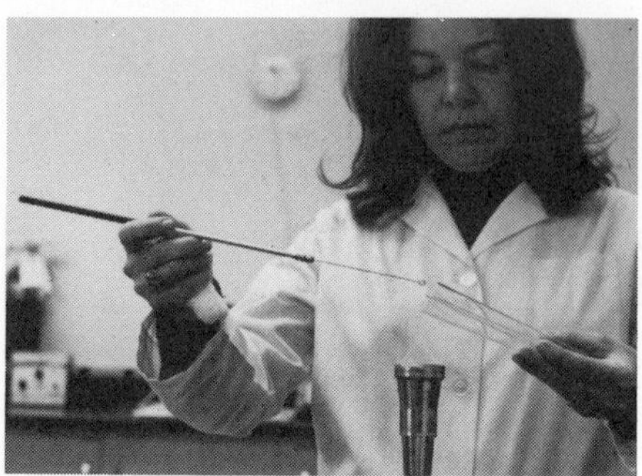

5. This figure shows positions of both hands and the way the needle is passed through the flame.

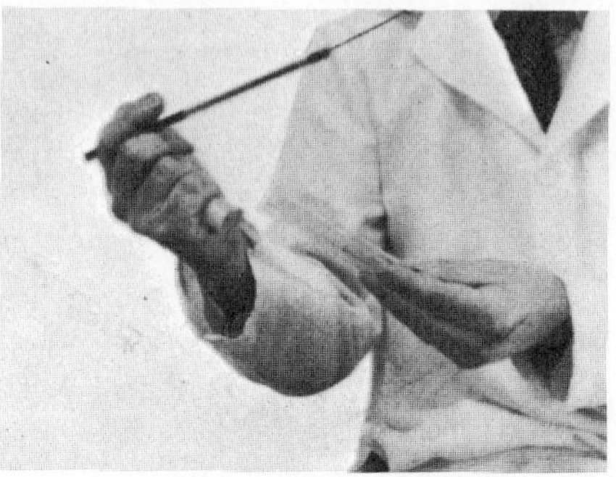

6. The caps are lifted from the test tubes with the left hand as shown.

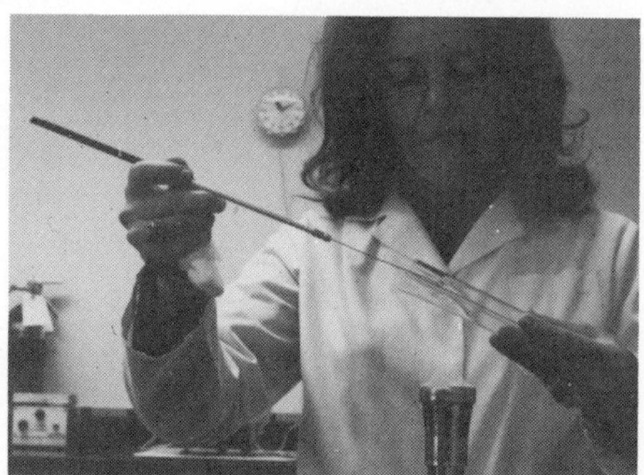

7. The inoculating needle is inserted into the tube containing the bacterial culture. It is then passed into the sterile tube to the fresh medium. The needle holder must not touch the inside of the tubes, since any unflamed part of the needle contaminates any surface it touches. Please note the straight line from one hand to the other, resulting when tubes are properly inoculated.

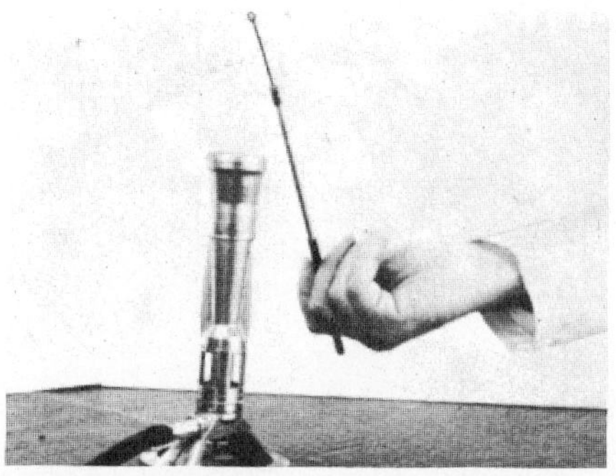

8. After the caps have been replaced on the tubes, the needle is flamed as shown. This is done from the holder toward the loop on the needle, to prevent splatter.

Laboratory Exercise 5

TOPIC: SIZE RELATIONSHIPS OF BACTERIA TO SOME OTHER BIOLOGICAL MATERIALS

OBJECTIVES:
1. To give the student experience in the use of a compound microscope and the oil immersion lens.
2. To show size relationships of bacteria with common objects. (Compare with Exercises 3, 4 and 6.)

EQUIPMENT:
1. A compound microscope.
2. Immersion oil (Crown, Cargill's, Shillaber's, or equal quality, but *not* a mineral oil.
3. *Prepared slides* of bacteria showing bacilli, cocci, spirilli, spores, flagella, capsules, and so on.
4. Prepared slides of human red blood cells.
5. Toothpicks.
6. Clean glass slides (clean with cleansing powder, if necessary).
7. Clean coverslips.
8. Aqueous methylene blue.

Procedure:

KEY STEPS	IMPORTANT POINTS
1. With the high dry power objective in position, focus on the slides listed under **Equipment.**	1.1. You will not be able to see enough detail with ×430 magnification.
2. Change to the oil immersion objective. (See directions under focusing a microscope.	2.1. Because bacteria are so small, the best magnification for examining them is obtained by using the oil immersion objective.
3. Carefully examine the slides and make drawings of your observations in the spaces provided.	3.1. Note similarities and differences among the slides you examine. 3.2. In your drawings show differences of size, shape, and any unusual structures. 3.3. Note the differences in size between the red blood cells on the prepared slide and the bacterial strains examined.
4. With a forceps pull out one hair from your head. Examine with low and high dry magnification.	4.1. Note that dark hairs are usually thicker than light hairs and that curly hairs are flat, but straight hairs are round. What does a dyed hair look like?
5. Place a drop of tap water on a clean glass slide. With a toothpick, remove material from between your teeth and on the surface of your gums. Place this material in the drop of water and cover with a coverslip. Examine with low and high dry magnification.	5.1. The water provides for dilution of the material scraped from your teeth and gums. 5.2. The coverslip protects the lenses of the objectives. 5.3. You will be able to see more detail on this material by using two magnifications. 5.4. This is similar to one of the early experiments that were performed by Antony van Leeuwenhoek.

<table>
<tr><td align="center">KEY STEPS</td><td align="center">IMPORTANT POINTS</td></tr>
<tr><td>6. After examining the slide prepared in step 5, place a drop of methylene blue under the coverslip. Allow to stand for 5 min. Reexamine the slide.</td><td>6.1. The stain will show structures you were unable to see without the stain.</td></tr>
</table>

Record of Results:

1. Draw what you observed on the slides with low and high dry power magnification. Try to show relative size differences under these magnifications. Show as much detail as possible in your drawing from the slide prepared from teeth scrapings.
2. Label each drawing with the name of the substance and the magnification (Ex.: ×100, ×440, ×970).

Drawings of Size Relationships of Bacteria to Other Biologic Materials

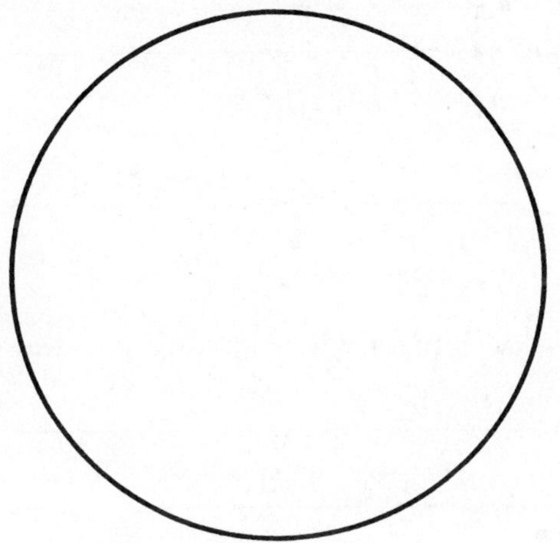

Figure 5–1. Object _______________

   Magnification × _______

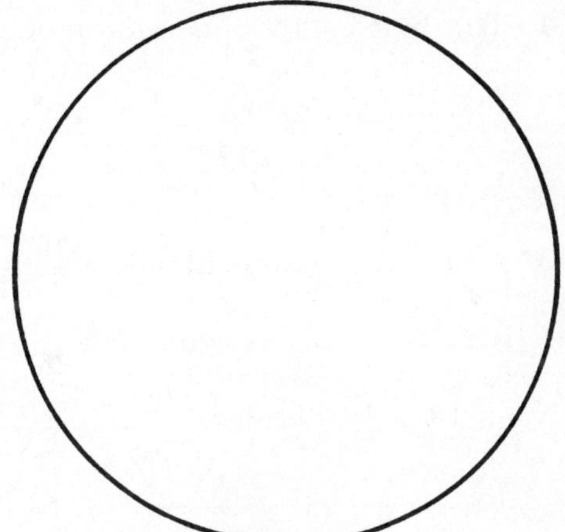

Figure 5–2. Object _______________

   Magnification × _______

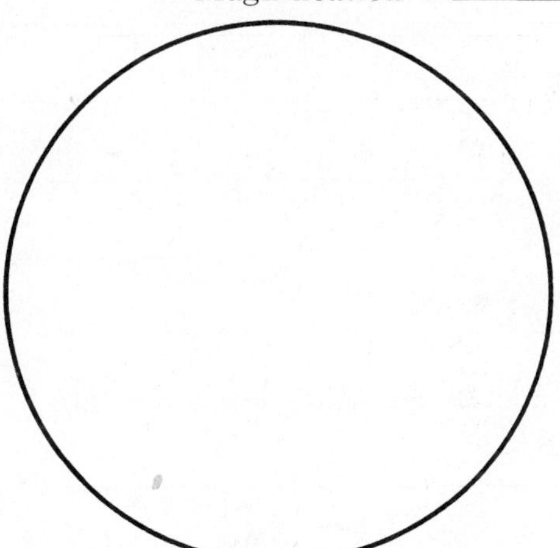

Figure 5–3. Object _______________

   Magnification × _______

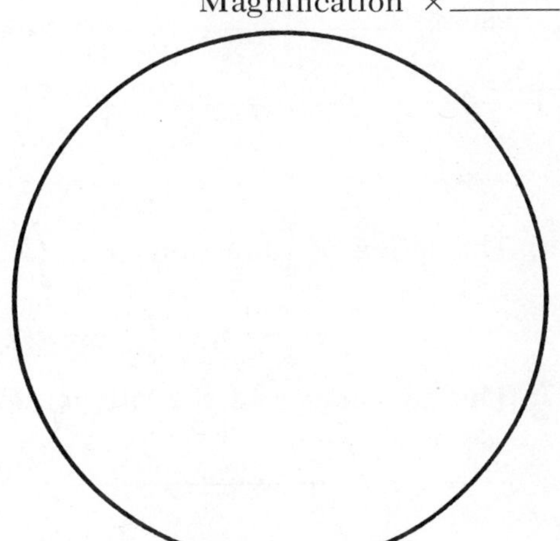

Figure 5–4. Object _______________

   Magnification × _______

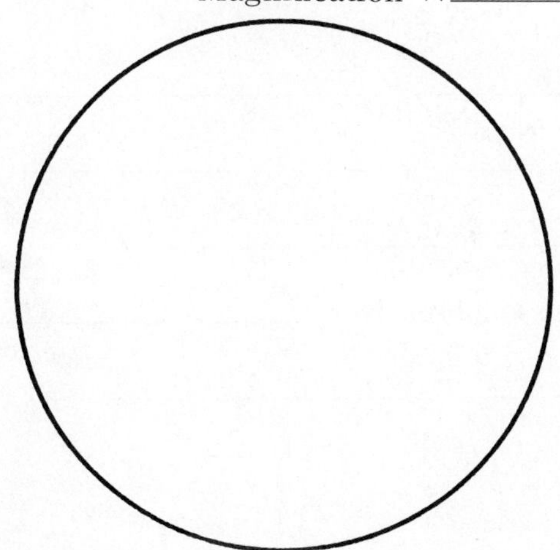

Figure 5–5. Object _______________

   Magnification × _______

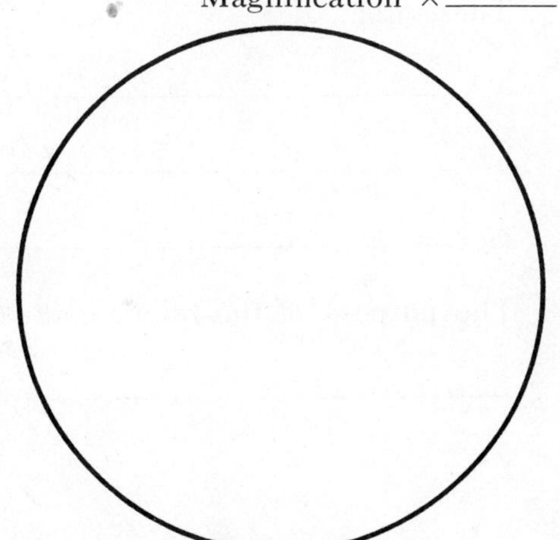

Figure 5–6. Object _______________

   Magnification × _______

Questions:

1. The first compound microscope was made by _______________________

   in __________(year).

2. A micrometer (μm) is _______________________

3. A red blood cell is almost exactly __________ μm in size.

4. It is essential that you always focus away from the object when looking into the

   microscope because _______________________

   ____

5. It is essential that you always look into the microscope with both eyes open be-

   cause _______________________

   ____

   ____

6. The index of refraction is _______________________

   ____

7. The advantages of the oil immersion objective over the other objectives are _

   ____

   ____

8. Morphologically, bacteria are classified into three distinct main groups.
   These are:

   a. _______________________

   b. _______________________

   c. _______________________

9. The purpose of the oil in using an oil immersion lens is _______________________

   ____

10. Name three morphologic structures seen on some of the prepared slides and give

your description of each.

a. ____

b. ____

c. ____

Laboratory Exercise 6

TOPIC: MORPHOLOGY OF PROTOZOA AND BACTERIA IN HANGING DROPS

OBJECTIVES:
1. To help the student understand the structure and motility of microscopic protozoa and note the much smaller size of the bacteria.
2. To help the student understand the similarities and differences in structure, method of obtaining food, and movement of microscopic protozoa.
3. To show the difference between true motility of bacteria and brownian movement.

EQUIPMENT:
1. Commercial liquid culture of any species of *Ameba*.
2. Commercial liquid culture of any species of *Paramecium*.
3. Sample of stagnant pond water if possible with protozoa and algae.
4. 24 hr broth culture of *Staphylococcus aureus* (nonpathogenic strain) or *Staphylococcus epidermidis*.
5. 24 hr broth culture of *Bacillus subtilis*.
6. 24 hr broth culture of *Escherichia coli*.
7. Clean hollow-ground glass slides.
8. Clean coverslips.
9. Either 5% Lysol, 5% phenol solution, or saponated solution of cresol in a large beaker.

Procedure:

KEY STEPS	IMPORTANT POINTS
1. Follow the procedure outlined in the Laboratory Exercise 4, Steps 1 to 13. Note: Allow the hanging drop slide of *Ameba* to lie undisturbed on the laboratory desk for a few minutes.	1.1. Amebas move more slowly than paramecia. Why? ____________________________ 1.2. What is the mode of movement of amebas? ____________________________ of paramecia? ____________________________ ____________________________ 1.3. Note different kinds of microorganisms in the pond water. Perhaps you can see some algae? 1.4. How would you tell whether they could be considered to be a plant or an animal? ____________________________
2. Using the bacterial cultures listed, prepare a hanging drop on a coverslip as described in Exercise 4.	2.1. See Exercise 4.

KEY STEPS	**IMPORTANT POINTS**
3. Examine the slides under high dry power.	3.1. Bacteria are so small that you cannot see them under low power magnification. 3.2. It is easier to observe hanging drop preparations by focusing on the edge of the drop with the light considerably reduced. The big droplets you see on the outside of the drop are water of condensation. Bacteria are best seen on the inner edge of the drop. 3.3. Don't forget to look for true motility and for brownian movement.
4. Discard each slide in the solution of disinfectant.	4.1. You should not separate the coverslip from the slide before placing them in the disinfectant solution. 4.2. Remember that you are working with living bacteria, one of which can produce infection (*Staphylococcus aureus*). 4.3. If you should accidentally break a coverglass which has a viable culture on it, report this accident *immediately* to your instructor. Do you remember how to use Lysol properly to disinfect?

Record of Results:

1. Draw an *Ameba* under high power (on the next page).
2. Show pseudopods and direction of flow of protoplasm.
3. Draw a *Paramecium* under high power (on the next page).
4. Draw a picture of another microorganism you saw in pond water, perhaps an alga.
5. Make drawings of the bacteria seen and record in spaces provided (on the next page).
6. Record which organisms showed true motility and which organisms showed brownian movement (on the next page).

Drawings of Organisms Seen in Hanging Drop

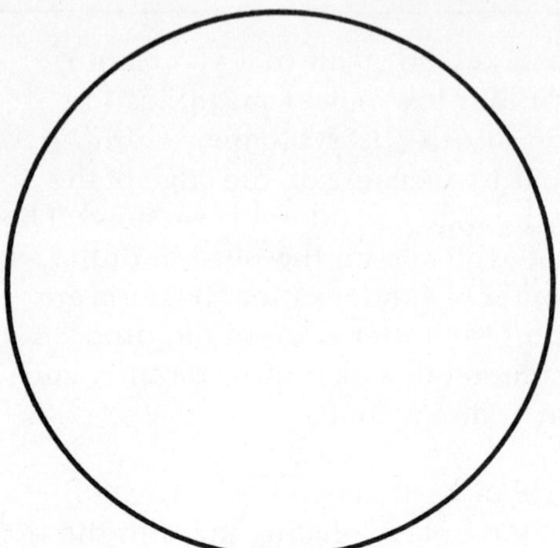

Figure 6–1. Object *Ameba*

Magnification ×________

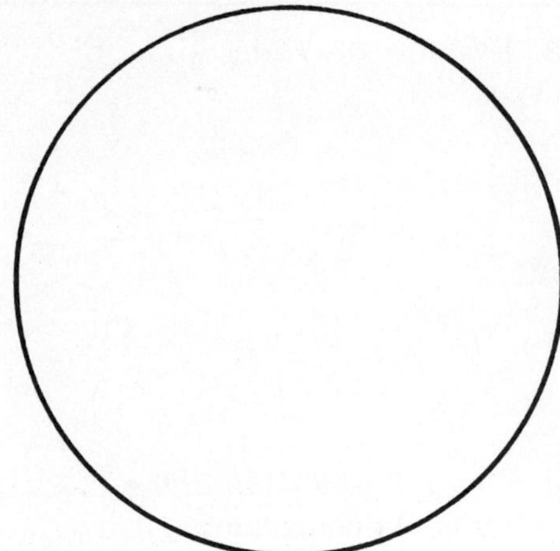

Figure 6–2. Object *Paramecium*

Magnification ×________

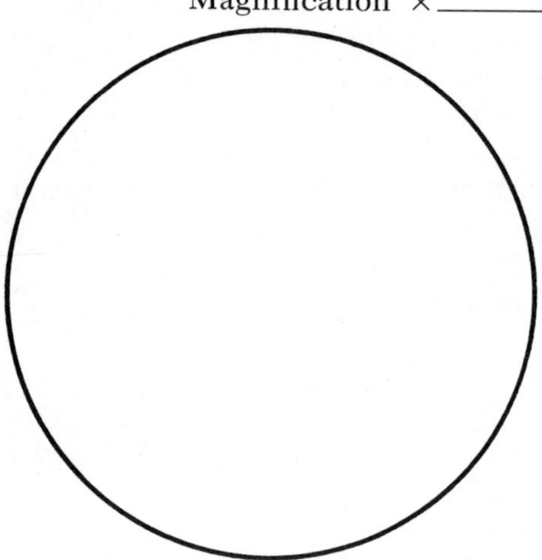

Figure 6–3. Object________________

Magnification ×________

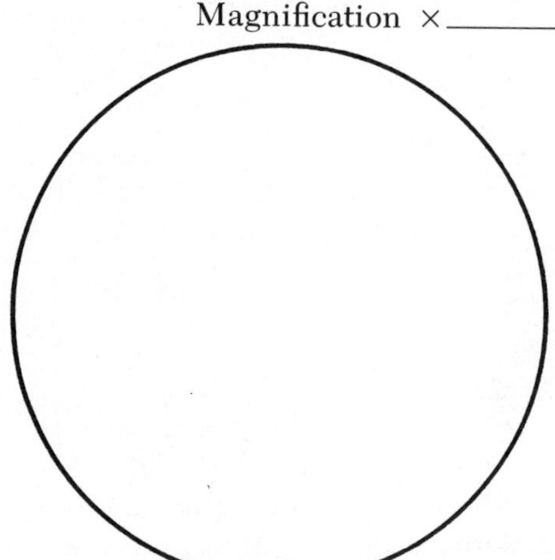

Figure 6–4. Object________________

Magnification ×________

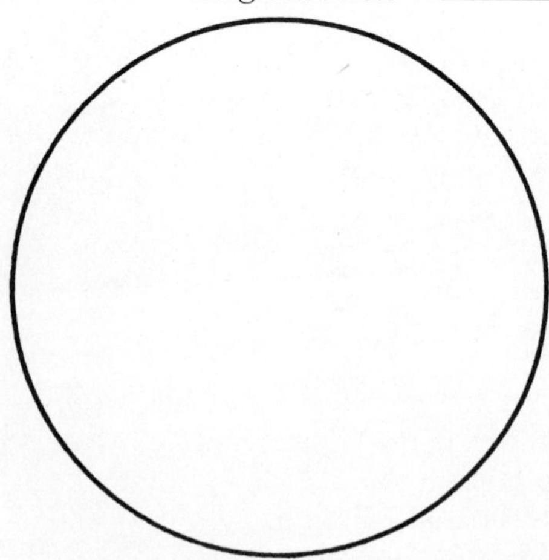

Figure 6–5. Object________________

Magnification ×________

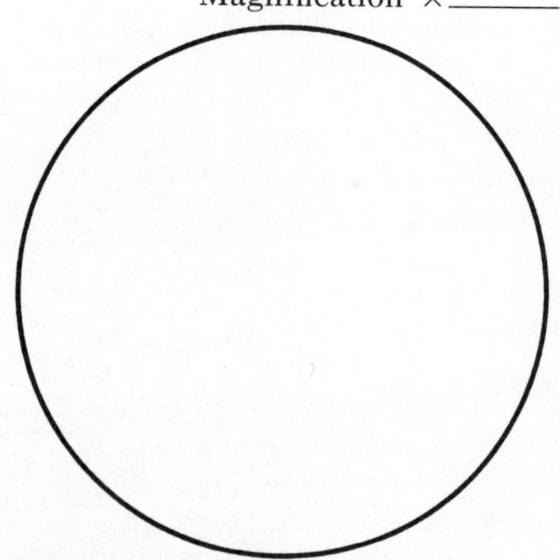

Figure 6–6. Object________________

Magnification ×________

Questions:

1. What are the similarities and differences in the structure, motility and methods of obtaining food of an *Ameba* and a *Paramecium*?

Similarities	Differences

2. Define: a. True motility _______________________________________

         b. Brownian movement _______________________________________

3. Organisms which display true motility probably have _______________________

    which are microscopic organs of _______________________________________

4. Different types of flagellation are _______________ , _______________ ,

    _______________ and _______________________________________

TOPIC: THE CARE AND HANDLING OF GLASSWARE IN A MICROBIOLOGY LABORATORY

In microbiology all glassware must be chemically clean and sterile, if pure cultures are to be maintained. This means that glassware must be thoroughly washed, rinsed with tap water, and then rinsed in distilled water before medium is added, or dry glassware is sterilized. Sometimes a cleaning solution is necessary for adequate cleansing of pipettes and other tubes too small to be cleaned with a brush. Cleaning solution can be made by putting 40 g of potassium dichromate in a tall glass cylinder and adding 800 ml of 25% sulfuric acid. *(This must be used with caution.)* Pipettes should remain in the cylinder overnight and be washed with tap water and rinsed with distilled water the next morning. Be sure that rinsing is adequate.

No cracked glassware should be used. These cracks, if present, may contaminate your cultures and spoil your results.

Dry glassware is usually sterilized in the hot air oven. Liquids and agar media in glassware are autoclaved. Petri dishes may be wrapped in paper in sets of two or three or may be stacked in cylinders or trays. They are sterilized in the hot air oven (at 170–180 C) for 2 to 3 hr. Pipettes may be wrapped in paper or put in cylinders and sterilized in the hot air oven at 170–180 C for 2 hr. Sterile disposable Petri dishes and sterile disposable pipettes are available at a reasonable cost. Use of these disposable items may prove to be less expensive than purchase of glass ones because of the costs of cleaning and sterilizing. This is certainly true for disposable syringes and needles, neatly and practically packed to assure sterility.

Cotton plugs for tubes are made with nonabsorbent cotton. The plugs should be firm enough to support the weight of the tube when suspended by the plugs. Cotton plugs in test tubes allow the free passage of air into and from the tubes but prevent the entrance of microorganisms. Cotton plugs should always remain dry. A wet cotton plug is a likely source of contamination. Your laboratory instructor will demonstrate the proper way of "rolling a plug." Now, however, the tubes are often closed with loose fitting plastic or metal caps. These can be properly washed and autoclaved and thus are reusable.

If glassware must be sterilized in the autoclave, the temperature is maintained at 121 C (15 lb pressure per square inch*) for 15 to 20 min. In 18 lb pressure autoclaves the temperature may go up to 124.5 C and the time required to sterilize can be correspondingly reduced to be 6 to 10 min. The autoclave is not the instrument of choice for dry glassware, but is the instrument of choice for media and all solutions that must be sterilized. As sterilizers which use microbicidal gases become more readily available, these may replace or supplement the conventional steam autoclave.

TOPIC: PREPARATION OF CULTURE MEDIA

All of the media suggested for use in this laboratory manual can be prepared successfully by using commercially prepared dehydrated media and following the directions given on the packages. In some instances, carbohydrates are added to the broth or agar base. Indicators may be added to the media as needed in certain exercises. Packages of pre-weighed media† are currently available and very convenient to use.

The author uses 10 mm × 75 mm tubes for broth cultures and slants. These tubes conserve media, are convenient for students to use, and fit more easily into the space in the incubator and refrigerator.

In preparing nutrient agar medium for plating, it may be convenient to tube the medium in 15 to 20 ml amounts. This provides enough agar medium to cover the bottom of the Petri dishes ordinarily used in the laboratory. In another method, the flask with the sterile liquid hot agar medium is kept in a 65 C water bath until it is convenient to pour the plates (see the next experiment).

The most commonly used media are nutrient broth and nutrient agar and some modifications of both. Other media will be mentioned later on in this laboratory manual.

NUTRIENT BROTH

```
Meat extract...................... 3 g
Peptone .......................... 10 g
Distilled water  ............. 1,000 ml
```

Dissolve the ingredients in the distilled water. Adjusting to pH 7.2 with 1 N NaOH, dispense in test tubes. Sterilize in the autoclave.

NUTRIENT AGAR

To make nutrient agar from nutrient broth add 2% Bacto Agar-Agar (Difco Agar) to the broth (20 g/liter).

---

*Often written as 15 psi.
†Fisher Scientific Co., Chicago, Ill.

MODERN METHODS

It is not practical any more to boil beef to make beef extract, to weigh out peptone, or to make an infusion broth. Usually one follows the label on a bottle of "Nutrient Broth" powder prepared by Difco Laboratories, BBL (formerly Baltimore Biological Laboratory), or Fisher Scientific Co. The label states the composition of the medium in the bottle and how much of the powder should be weighed out to give 1 liter of medium with distilled water. This is usually 8 g per liter.

Dehydrated solid media like Nutrient Agar are usually too soft for southern temperatures. If the label on this bottle says 15 g agar, an extra 5 g Agar Agar (Difco Agar) needs to be added for this medium to become hard enough.

TOPIC: THE RELATIONS OF STERILE TECHNIQUE IN MICROBIOLOGY TO CLINICAL MEDICAL APPLICATIONS

There is a direct and specific relationship between sterile technique in microbiology and many clinical (hospital) procedures. In microbiology sterile media are used. These media are most frequently sterilized in culture tubes. In addition, sterile Petri dishes for receiving sterile nutrient agar media, sterile pipettes for accurately measuring some solutions, sterile inoculating needles for transfer of specific organisms from one place to another, sterile applicators for culturing certain materials, and sterile water for making dilutions are also used routinely. These materials may be sterilized either by autoclaving (15 lb steam at 121 C for 15 to 30 min, or less in high pressure autoclaves), in germicidal gas sterilizers, or in the direct flame (used for inoculating needles). Preferably, dry materials are sterilized in a hot air oven at 170 to 180 C for 2 to 3 hr.

Forceps tips are dipped into alcohol and passed through the flame so that the alcohol burns in the air and the forceps tips become sterile. These sterile forceps (tip only) are referred to as transfer forceps. This is a quick method of sterilization and quite effective when objects are to be transferred under sterile conditions.

In microbiology, conscientious attempts are made to keep sterile Petri dishes free from contaminating organisms until sterile agar medium is put in them. Then the cover of the Petri dish is raised only as far as necessary to pour the medium into the bottom of the dish. The cover is always held with the inside down to prevent organisms from the air from falling into the inside. The cover is always replaced as quickly as possible after agar is poured. The inoculating loop is sterilized in the direct flame and not allowed to touch anything until it is used to transfer material from a specific source. Then the material is transferred either to media or to a glass slide and the inoculating loop resterilized by heating in a direct flame. This is done to prevent transfer of material to undesirable places, i.e., materials which need to be kept sterile, and your desk, hands and books. In other words, know where the microorganisms are and keep them from being contaminated by anything. Remember that microorganisms are everywhere—on your hands, in the air, on all surfaces. Nothing except living tissue protected from the outside environment is free from microorganisms unless it has been made aseptic.

In the laboratory and in hospitals, procedures are carried out to try to keep sterile objects free from contaminating organisms. Sterile dressings are either wrapped in muslin or kept in metal containers. These sterile dressings must be handled only with sterile instruments. In order to carry out sterile technique successfully in laboratories and hospitals, it is important to remember that microorganisms are everywhere, except on surfaces that have been sterilized and have been kept sterile. As in microbiology, covers should be held with the inside down to prevent microorganisms from the air from contaminating the inside sterile surface. Covers should be left off containers only for sufficient time to remove, or put in, sterile material. Sterile instruments should touch only sterile objects to keep them sterile. If instruments have been contaminated, they should be resterilized.

In caring for a patient with a specific infection, attempts are made to keep the infection confined. Therefore, special precautions are used when bringing contaminated materials from the area where these patients are isolated. These materials must be made free of the specific organism before the materials can be used for other patients. In reverse precautions used with debilitated patients, patients who have had open-heart surgery and premature infants, all materials or objects are sterile or as clean as possible. The problem in these cases is to prevent any infectious organism from invading a patient. As in microbiology, know where microorganisms are, keep sterile materials free from contamination, and destroy microorganisms in the patient and on contaminated areas.

Laboratory Exercise 7

TOPIC: POURING AND INOCULATING AGAR PLATES

OBJECTIVES:
1. To give the student experience in pouring and inoculating sterile agar plates.
2. To give the student additional understanding of the principles of aseptic or sterile technique.

EQUIPMENT:
1. Sterile Petri dishes (plates) (two or more).
2. Sterile tubes of nutrient agar (two or more), or sterile Erlenmeyer flasks, half filled with nutrient agar.
3. Sterile cotton applicators (dry and moist).*
4. A nutrient agar slant culture of red pigmented *Serratia marcescens* (or another selected bacterial culture).

Procedure:

KEY STEPS	IMPORTANT POINTS
1. Heat tubes of nutrient agar in a water bath or beaker of water until the agar is completely liquefied. The nutrient agar may also be autoclaved in Erlenmeyer flasks and kept in a water bath at 65 C until needed for use.	1.1. Agar melts at about 97 C and remains liquid until cooled to 40 C. Once solidified it must be reheated to 97 C to cause its liquefaction. The nutrient agar may be kept in a 65 C water bath for several hours before use.
2. Cool the tubes or Erlenmeyer flasks to about 50 C.	2.1. Allow tubes of nutrient agar to cool in the beaker, or the flasks from the water bath, at room temperature to about 45 C. 2.2. Do not add cold water to the beaker because the agar on the sides of the tube may solidify 2.3. While agar does not liquefy until it is heated to 90 to 100 C, it does not resolidify until it cools to approximately 40 C.
3. Place sterile Petri dishes on the laboratory table by sliding them on, cover side up.	3.1. Do not attempt to unstack the Petri dishes on the table by lifting them; instead slide each dish carefully to spread them on the table. If the cover is lifted even slightly, air currents which carry dust will enter and be a source of possible contamination of the plates.

---

*If cotton applicators are sterilized in a large test tube (10 to 12 in a tube), a small amount of water can be added to the bottom of the tube and the tube can then be autoclaved. This provides moist cotton applicators which can be used over dry surfaces.

KEY STEPS	IMPORTANT POINTS
4. When the agar has cooled to 50 C, remove the cotton stopper from the tube; flame the mouth of the agar tube; raise the cover of the sterile Petri dish enough to get the mouth of the tube in and pour the sterile agar into the dish. The procedure is the same when an Erlenmeyer flask is used.	4.1. The mouth of the tube must be flamed because you are going to pour sterile medium over it. This flaming should be sufficient to destroy the microorganisms on the lip of the tube. 4.2. When an Erlenmeyer flask is used to pour the nutrient agar into the Petri dishes, the cotton plug is placed into another sterile Petri dish to avoid contamination of the sterile part of the plug, and the mouth of the flask is flamed between each pouring; many dishes may be filled from one flask. Your instructor may come around and pour your plates when they are positioned at the edge of the table. 4.3. Raising the Petri dish cover only slightly keeps the nutrient agar protected from air contamination.
5. Return the cover of the Petri dish to its original position; gently rotate the dish so that the agar covers the entire surface of the bottom.	5.1. When you are rotating the Petri dish, be sure that the agar does not go over the side. This will result in having the cover stick to the bottom and may result in contamination.
6. Put the dish in an undisturbed place to harden the medium.	6.1. By leaving the agar plate undisturbed, you will have a smooth surface to inoculate. 6.2. The agar will harden in about 15 to 20 min at ordinary room temperature.

Rather complicated ways of streaking an agar plate have been devised by many microbiologists. The purpose is always the same: to redistribute bacteria from the loop needle onto the plate in such a way that "isolated cells" are deposited on a part of the plate. These isolated cells give rise to isolated *pure colonies. Any method that results in pure colonies* and no contamination after streaking a plate *is acceptable.*

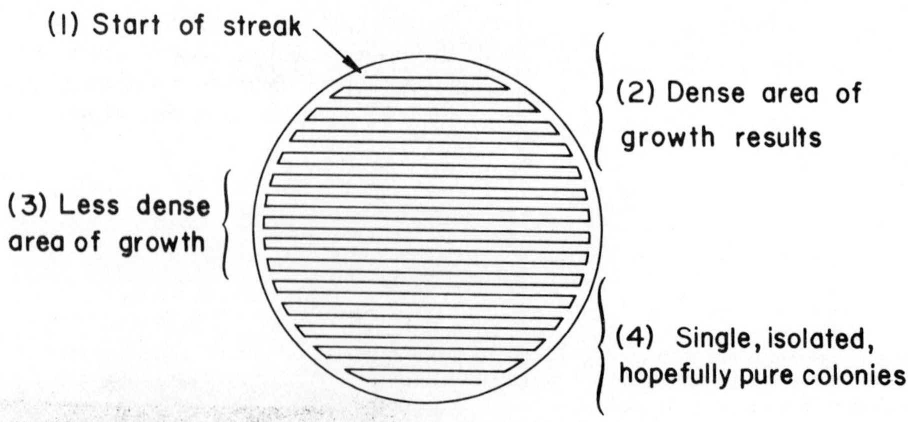

Perhaps the simplest way to streak a plate is to leave it on the table, raise the top with the left hand and streak as **_close as possible_** rapidly from one end of the plate to the other. If done properly, the lower half of the streaked plate will contain isolated colonies after incubation.

There are many ways to streak a plate. The purpose is to obtain isolated colonies, the progenies of single cells distributed in a section on the nutrient agar surface. For this reason it is best to streak as near together as possible in long close strokes. Some workers pick up a Petri plate to streak it; this is objectionable since microorganisms may thus be brought close to the face, the mouth and the eyes.

In a very recent method, a drop containing the inoculum is placed in the center of a Petri plate, the cover is put on and the plate is rotated on a centrifuge-like device at the right speed to distribute individual cells toward the periphery, where subsequently isolated colonies develop. If this procedure is done correctly, most of the plate will contain evenly distributed single colonies.

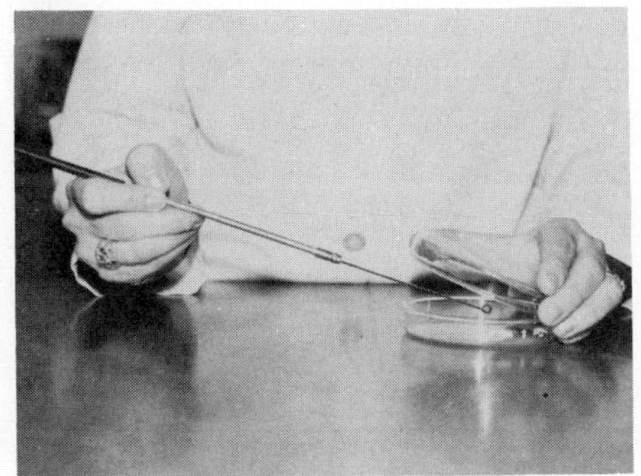

KEY STEPS	**IMPORTANT POINTS**
7. Inoculate the agar plate in the way previously illustrated: a. Obtain culture material *(Serratia marcescens)* from the tube on a flamed sterile inoculating loop; raise the cover of the Petri dish enough to permit entrance of the loop and streak the plate in the way diagrammed. b. If inoculating from a moist surface in the environment (e.g., throat or tonsils), use a dry sterile applicator (swab) to obtain the material and use the same technique as in 7a. c. If inoculating from a dry surface in the environment (e.g., skin, surface of the table), use a sterile moist cotton applicator to obtain the material and use the same technique as in 7a.	7.1. Do not dig up the agar. 7.2. The surface of the agar should be smooth when you are finished. The inculating loop should barely touch the surface of the agar and not penetrate it. Some workers advise picking up the agar-containing portion of the plate and streaking it in the air, at face level. This is most undesirable and dangerous, since all bacteria must be considered potentially infective. 7.3. You may read over the directions in Exercise 4 and look at the illustrations for the proper technique of getting microorganisms from cultures into new test tubes.
8. Label all plates on the bottom.	8.1. Labels should include your initials, the source of the material and the date. 8.2. By labeling on the bottom, you make certain that the bottom of the Petri plate that contains the organisms also shows the right label.

<table>
<tr><td align="center">**KEY STEPS**</td><td align="center">**IMPORTANT POINTS**</td></tr>
</table>

	8.3. You may need to look through the cover to see if the culture has grown, although for your *final* reading you always remove the cover for a *short time* to see and/or count the colonies.
9. Incubate all plates in an inverted position in your desk or in an incubator (consult your instructor) until the next laboratory period.	9.1. Plates usually must be incubated upside down because water of condensation may form on the cover, drop on the growth and spread over the surface of the agar. This destroys discrete colonies. 9.2. Most of the organisms in the environment will grow at ordinary room temperatures. Bacterial human pathogens prefer 35 to 37 C, the usual incubator temperature.

Record of Results:

1. After the Petri plates have been incubated, record the amount and the kind of growth. Describe the size and the shape of the colonies, using appropriate terms such as small, round, spreading, irregular, punctiform, smooth, rhizoid, large, and so on. Describe the color of the colonies and their consistency, i.e., smooth, crumbly, caseous, butyrous, and so on.
2. Draw typical colonies. (See pages 201 and 202 in Appendix for examples.)

GROWTH OF COLONIES ON NUTRIENT AGAR PLATES*

Source of Culture	Amount of Growth	Shape of Colonies	Color	Consistency of Colonies	Drawings of Typical Colonies

*Incubate at 37 C for 24 hr.

Questions:

1. Agar medium liquefies at __________ temperature. It resolidifies at ______________ temperature. This is advantageous because ____

____

2. The cover of a Petri dish is rarely completely removed except for special duties

because ____

____

3. The advantages of a nutrient agar culture in a Petri dish over a broth culture are ____

____

4. The advantages of a nutrient agar plate over a nutrient agar slant are _____________

____

5. The advantages of agar over gelatin are ____

____

6. The natural source of agar is ____

TOPIC: KNOWN RATIONALE FOR A SELECTED GROUP OF STAINING PROCEDURES
USED WITH BACTERIA

OBJECTIVES: 1. To help the student understand the rationale of staining procedures.
2. To introduce the student to the general purposes of certain methods of staining.

General Discussion:

Without methods of staining microorganisms, the microbiologist would know little about the cytologic structures found in the microbial world. All protoplasm (plant and animal, human and bacteria, protozoan and fungal) is colorless or slightly grey and is transparent. Organisms of the microbial world are so minute that they are difficult to see with the microscope unless they are colored with some type of dye. (It is amazing that Antony van Leeuwenhoek saw as much as he did without stains to increase the visibility of his "animalcules.") By staining microorganisms it is possible to see not only size and shape but also certain special structures such as spores, flagella, and granules, and also to demonstrate chemical factors which differentiate groups of microorganisms. In addition, dyes may be used in culture media to influence the growth of some members of the microbial world, often by inhibiting unwanted organisms. The discussion here will be limited to the use of dyes to observe size and shape and specific structure, and to examining chemical factors involved.

The dyes used by the microbiologist are synthetic derivatives of aniline (aniline dyes). Because basic dyes are attracted chemically to the constituents of nuclei, dyes which are chemical alkalis are most commonly used in staining microorganisms. Basic dyes give a uniform stain to bacterial cells. Note the use of sodium bicarbonate in the Gram stain to assure basic conditions.

Many workers have attempted to explain why stains are effective. In addition to the chemical theory just stated, a physical factor of adsorption may be important. The dye particles may be fixed to the cells because of opposite charges carried by the dye and protoplasm which would attract each other like positive and negative charges of electricity. However, even in this age of scientific knowledge, the exact physical and chemical mechanisms of staining bacteria are not wholly understood.

Categories of Staining:

1. *Simple Staining:* Any basic aniline dye may be used. The most frequent ones are methylene blue, eosin, safranine, basic fuchsin and crystal violet (also known as gentian violet). Use 0.05 g of methylene blue in 1,000 ml water; 0.5 g of safranine in 100 ml water; 0.1 g basic fuchsin in 100 ml water; and 1.0 g of crystal violet in 100 ml water.

2. *Differential Staining:*
   a. **Gram's Stain**—Modified Kopeloff and Beerman's Method.* The following solutions are used (prepared for you by your instructor or laboratory assistant):

Gentian Violet Solution

Gentian (crystal) violet .... 1 g
Water .... 100 ml

Sodium Bicarbonate Solution

Sodium bicarbonate .... 1 g
Water .... 20 ml

Iodine Solution

Potassium iodide .... 2 g
Iodine .... 1 g
Distilled water .... 300 ml

Mix the iodine and potassium iodide in a mortar and grind with a pestle until finely divided. Add distilled water in small portions to wash out the contents into a graduate cylinder. Finally add sufficient distilled water to make 300 ml. Mix well and

---

*Many different modifications of Gram's stain exist; this method is adapted from the one described by Williams, O.B., and Wyss, O.: Laboratory Manual for Elementary Bacteriology, 2nd Ed. 1949, Austin, Texas, Hemphill's.

if necessary filter through filter paper. (Some methods employ 10 ml normal NaOH in this solution.)

Decolorizing Agent (Acetone-Alcohol)

Alcohol, 95 per cent .... 7 parts
Acetone .... 3 parts

Counterstain

Basic fuchsin (or safranine, or Bismark brown). 0.1 g
Distilled water .... 100.0 ml

Technique. Use an 18 to 24 hr bacterial culture. Gram stains are easier to make from agar slants than broth cultures, but either may be used. Transfer a loopful of the organisms to a drop of water on the slant. Spread and let air-dry. Pass the dry film briefly through a flame, which fixes the film.

Stain the fixed film for about 3 min with the crystal violet solution made alkaline by adding a drop or two of the bicarbonate solution. Rinse with the iodine solution and allow to stand for about 2 min. Wash and destain with the acetone-alcohol mixture by allowing it to flow over the film, drop by drop, until the droppings show no tint of color (usually less than 10 sec). Wash and counterstain for about 30 sec with safranine or basic fuchsin. Wash, blot, or drain dry and examine under the oil immersion lens.

Most bacteria may be placed in one of two groups by the reaction to the Gram stain. If the organism retains the violet stain it is recorded as gram-positive. Gram-negative organisms lose the violet stain under treatment with the acetone-alcohol mixture and are stained red by the counterstain. The Gram reaction is variable with age and should be done on cultures 18 to 24 hr old for most reliable results.

Laboratory Exercise 9 also gives details of procedure for the Gram stain.

A partial list of the common pathogenic bacteria is given, with the reaction of each to the Gram stain.

Gram-positive:	*Gram-negative:*
Actinomyces species	*Enterobacter (Aerobacter) aerogenes*
Bacillus anthracis	*Brucella abortus*
Clostridium botulinum	*Brucella melitensis*
Clostridium tetani	*Brucella suis*
Clostridium perfringens (welchii)	*Haemophilus influenzae*
Corynebacterium diphtheriae	*Bordetella (Haemophilus) pertussis*
Streptococcus (Diplococcus) pneumoniae	*Neisseria gonorrhoeae*
Streptococcus hemolyticus	*Neisseria meningitidis*
Mycobacterium leprae	*Francisella (Pasteurella) tularensis*
Mycobacterium tuberculosis	*Yersinia (Pasteurella) pestis*
Staphylococcus aureus	*Pseudomonas aeruginosa*
Staphylococcus epidermidis (albus)	*Salmonella paratyphi*
	Salmonella typhi (typhosa)
	Shigella dysenteriae
	Vibrio cholerae (comma)

THEORIES ADVANCED TO EXPLAIN THE MECHANISM OF THE GRAM STAIN.

A. *Principle of the Gram Stain*
1. The initial stain stains practically all bacteria.
2. The iodine is a mordant which fixes the stain in gram-positive organisms.
3. The organisms which are decolorized by acetone-alcohol are gram-negative.
4. Gram-negative organisms will take the counterstain, usually red, but gram-positive bacteria will remain violet.

B. *Knaysi's Theory*
1. Gram-positive material absorbs more of the initial stain than does gram-negative material, and holds it more firmly.
2. When the mordant is added, a compound is formed that is insoluble in water and sparingly soluble in the decolorizing agent.
3. The rate at which the cell is decolorized is determined by the quantity of this precipitate formed in the cell and by the permeability of the cell wall to the dye-mordant complex. Gram-positive cells will be decolorized more slowly.

C. *Churchman's Theory*
1. Certain gram-positive bacteria consist of a gram-negative medulla which is surrounded by a gram-positive cortex.
2. The gram-positivity of an organism is attributed to the presence of the cortex, since in its absence the organism is gram-negative.

D. *Other Explanations*
1. Gram-positivity is due to the presence of unsaturated fatty acids which have a high affinity for iodine.
2. Gram-positivity is due to differences in permeability of the cell wall.

---

    b. **Acid-fast Stain.** Carbolfuchsin (steamed into the organism for three to five minutes), acid alcohol and methylene blue are used in succession. This method divides bacteria into two groups: acid-fast (those which retain the carbolfuchsin in spite of treatment with acid alcohol), and nonacid-fast (those which are decolorized by acid alcohol and have the color of the counterstain). Members of the genus *Mycobacterium* are acid-fast.

3. ***Stains for Specific Structures of Bacteria:***
    a. **Capsule Stain.** Crystal violet and copper sulfate are used. This stain shows capsules as halos around the bacteria.
    b. **Flagella Stain.** Ammonium alum, tannic acid, alcohol, basic fuchsin and methylene blue are used in succession. This stain depends on coating the flagella with sufficient material to make them visible.
    c. **Metachromatic Granule Stain.** Toluidine blue, methyl green, acetic acid, alcohol and Gram's iodine are used in succession. This stain shows the presence of volutin granules in some bacterial cells and is used most frequently for aiding in the identification of ***Corynebacterium diphtheriae.***
    d. **Spore Stain.** Carbolfuchsin (steamed on the smear), aqueous sodium sulfite and methylene blue are used in succession. With this stain, spores can be differentiated from vegetative cells.
    e. New staining techniques may replace those just listed, but for the purposes of this manual these new techniques will not be discussed.

Laboratory Exercise 8

TOPIC: SIMPLE STAINING

OBJECTIVES:
1. To introduce the student to simple staining.
2. To facilitate visualizing microorganisms for the student.
3. To give the student simple experience in bacteriologic techniques.

EQUIPMENT:
1. 24 hr broth cultures of *Bacillus subtilis*.
2. 24 hr broth cultures of *Staphylococcus aureus*.
3. 24 hr broth culture of *Enterobacter aerogenes*, or another gram-negative rod of choice.
4. Smears from gums of students.
5. Crystal violet (gentian violet).
6. Methylene blue.
7. Safranine.
8. Clean glass slides.
9. Slide holder.
10. Plastic wash bottle.

Procedure:

KEY STEPS	IMPORTANT POINTS
1. Clean all slides thoroughly and handle them by the edges only.	1.1. Dirt and fingerprints are magnified when looking at slides through the microscope. 1.2. Slides may be cleaned by mixing a few drops of water with Bon Ami and rubbing the surface of the slide with the lather. Let dry and polish with a clean cloth; do not put greasy fingers on the clean slide surfaces. Also remember that fat solvents like xylol or benzol remove oil.
2. Label the slides with the name of the microorganism.	2.1. Frequently several slides are made at one time and labels are essential to avoid errors in identification. 2.2. It is usually best to put this label on one end of the slide so that it does not become illegible with the stain, and the stain in the center of the slide. Good technique leaves the other end of the slide free for handling it on the microscope and the label is never covered with the stain. 2.3. One may write on the slide with a wax pencil or by using a gummed label. Never lick this label with your tongue or by moistening your fingers in your mouth. Why?.
3. Flame the inoculating loop and allow it to cool.	3.1. See Steps 3.1. and 3.2. in Exercise 4 and illustrations at end of Exercise 4 (Figure 4.4).

KEY STEPS	**IMPORTANT POINTS**
4. Remove the cotton plug or cap from the culture tube and obtain a loopful of the culture.	4.1. See Steps 4.1., 4.2., 4.3., 5.1., 5.2. in Exercise 4 and Figure 4–4.
5. Reinsert the cotton plug or cap.	5.1. See Step 6.1. in Exercise 4.
6. With the inoculating loop, spread a loopful of culture in a thin film in the center of the clean slide.	6.1. The culture may be a heavy growth of microorganisms. If you fail to make a thin film, the bacteria will be too close together to see them well. If you don't use enough of the organisms, you may not see any bacteria at all. For the beginner, it is usually best to get organisms from a slant rather (see Step 14) than from a liquid culture.
7. Flame the inoculating loop.	7.1. See Steps 3.1. and 8.2. in Exercise 4 and Figure 4–4.
8. Dry the film in the air. (This film is known as a smear.)	8.1. Drying the film removes the moisture, which facilitates staining. 8.2. Air-drying is preferable to heat-drying because it is important to avoid scorching the smear.
9. When the smear is completely dry, quickly pass the slide through the flame of the Bunsen burner three times. Keep the smear side of the slide up.	9.1. This process fixes the smear to the slide so that it is not as likely to wash off in the staining process. 9.2. Keeping the smear side up while passing it through the flame avoids scorching the smear.

10. Flood the center of the slide with one of the following stains for the time interval indicated:
     methylene blue   30–45 sec
     crystal violet   30–45 sec
     safranine   45–60 sec
	10.1. By flooding the smear on the slide, the cells are completely immersed in stain.
	 10.2. A time factor is essential to permit the stain to pass through the cell walls into the cells.

11. Wash the slide gently with tap water.	11.1. Gentle washing avoids washing off the smear. 11.2. This may be done by using a gentle stream of cold water from a plastic wash bottle. 11.3. The slide must be washed to remove the excess stain.

KEY STEPS	**IMPORTANT POINTS**
12. Dry the slide.	12.1. Slides may be dried by blotting between two pieces of paper towel or by drying in the air. 12.2. When blotting slides dry, be careful not to rub the smear. Rubbing will cause streaks and may remove the smear. 12.3. Slides cannot be examined with the oil immersion objective unless they are thoroughly dry.
13. Examine with the oil immersion objective.	13.1. Bacteria are seen best with the oil immersion lens. Do not waste your time using any other magnification.
14. When making a slide from an agar slant, place a drop of tap water on a clean slide; touch the sterile inoculating loop to the growth on the slant and mix this material thoroughly with some water from the drop. Then proceed as noted.	14.1. Growth on a slant is heavier than in a broth culture. Therefore, you need to dilute the suspension from the slant very thinly. 14.2. If you have barely touched the growth on the slant, you have thousands of bacteria. Thousands of microorganisms will not be visible to the naked eye but will be visible with the microscope.
15. With a sterile, cool inoculating loop, or cotton swab, make a smear from your gums and stain as just stated.	15.1 The smear from your gums will show human cells and food particles as well as bacteria.

Record of Results:

1. Make a drawing in color of each of the three organisms as observed with the oil immersion objective.
2. Make a drawing of the smear from the gums as observed with the oil immersion objective.

Questions:

1. Define each of the following terms:

   a. Smear (film)

   b. Fixing

   c. Culture

   d. Transfer

2. It is essential to use sterile bacteriologic techniques in removing material from

culture tubes because ____

____ .

3. Three reasons for staining bacteria are:

   a.

   b.

   c.

4. The inoculating loop is flamed before and after removing material from the culture

tube because ____

____

____ .

Drawings of Organisms Seen after Simple Staining

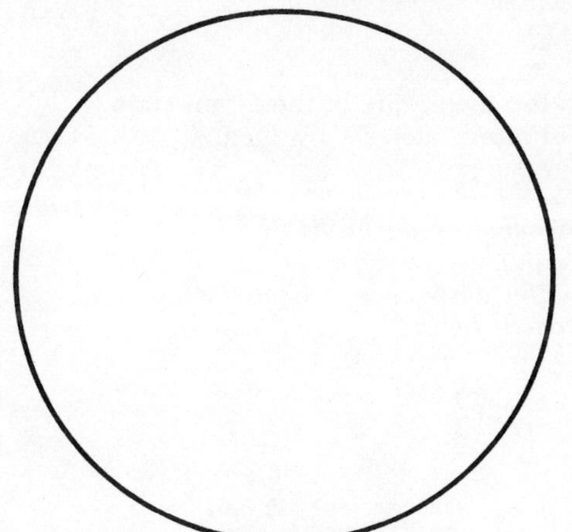

Figure 8–1. Object _______________

       Type of stain _________

       Magnification ×_________

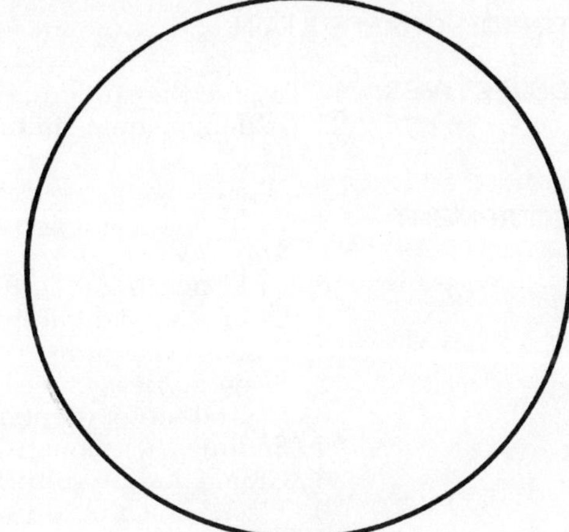

Figure 8–2. Object _______________

       Type of stain _________

       Magnification×_________

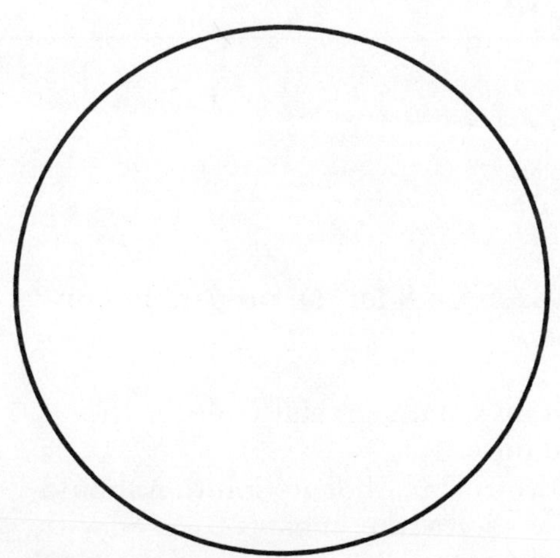

Figure 8–3. Object _______________

       Type of stain _________

       Magnification ×_________

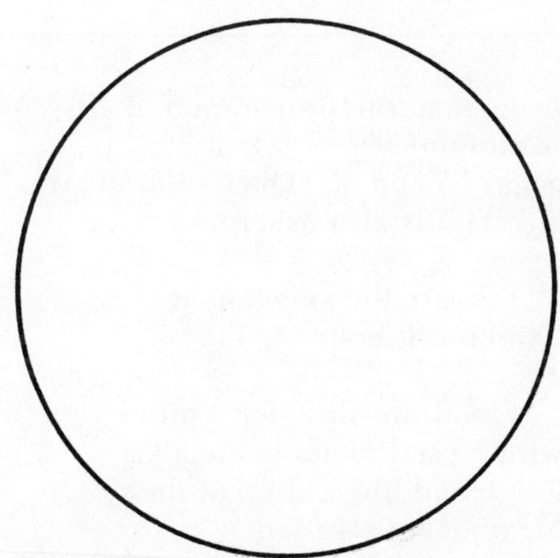

Figure 8–4. Object _______________

       Type of stain _________

       Magnification ×_________

Laboratory Exercise 9

TOPIC: GRAM'S STAIN

OBJECTIVES:
1. To give the student experience with the technique of the Gram stain.
2. To demonstrate methods of differentiating bacteria by means of the Gram stain.

EQUIPMENT:
1. 24 hr agar slant culture of *Staphylococcus epidermidis* or *Staphylococcus aureus* (nonpathogenic).
2. 24 hr agar slant culture of *Enterobacter aerogenes* or *Escherichia coli.*
3. 24 hr agar slant culture of *Streptococcus lactis.*
4. Smear from gums.
5. Slide holder.
6. Crystal violet (gentian violet).
7. Sodium bicarbonate solution.
8. Gram's iodine solution.
9. Plastic wash bottle with tap water.
10. Acetone alcohol solution.
11. Safranine or another counterstain.

Procedure:

KEY STEPS	IMPORTANT POINTS
1. Look at the preparation of all constituents for the Gram stain on pages 44 and 45. The technique of the stain is also described there.	
2. Prepare the smear as in Exercise 8, Step 14.	2.1. See Exercise 8 for the preparation of the smear.
3. Flood the slide for 3 min with crystal violet made alkaline by adding a drop of the bicarbonate solution.	3.1. In Gram's stain, crystal violet is the primary stain. 3.2. The drop of bicarbonate solution should be added as soon as the smear is covered with crystal violet.
4. Flood the slide for 2 min with Gram's iodine solution.	4.1. Gram's iodine is a mordant in this stain. 4.2. There is probably a chemical reaction which takes place between the primary stain, the mordant and the protoplasm of certain cells.
5. Wash the slide with tap water.	5.1. See Exercise 8, page 48.
6. Pour a few drops of acetone alcohol on the slide; tilt the slide from side to side to aid in washing; pour off the alcohol and repeat this process until no more dye flows from the smear.	6.1. Aniline dyes and iodine are both soluble in ethyl alcohol. Therefore, acetone alcohol can be used as a decolorizing agent. 6.2. You must guard against overdecolorizing the smear and also underdecolorizing.

KEY STEPS	IMPORTANT POINTS

7. Wash the slide with tap water from a wash bottle.

7.1. See Exercise 8, page 48.

8. Flood the slide for 30 sec to 1 min with safranine or another counterstain of your choice.

8.1. In this staining procedure, safranine is the counterstain.
8.2. While all cells will be stained with the counterstain, only those cells which have lost the crystal violet will look red under the microscope. All gram-positive cells will look purple.

9. Wash the slide with tap water, blot dry and examine with the oil immersion lens under the microscope.

9.1. See Exercise 8, pages 48 and 49.

Record of Results:

1. Draw, in color, samples of each of the organisms you saw. Record the results obtained in the spaces provided. Indicate which organism is gram-positive and which is gram-negative.
2. Draw, in color, what you observed in the smear from the gums. Record the results obtained in the space provided. Indicate which organisms were gram-positive and which were gram-negative.

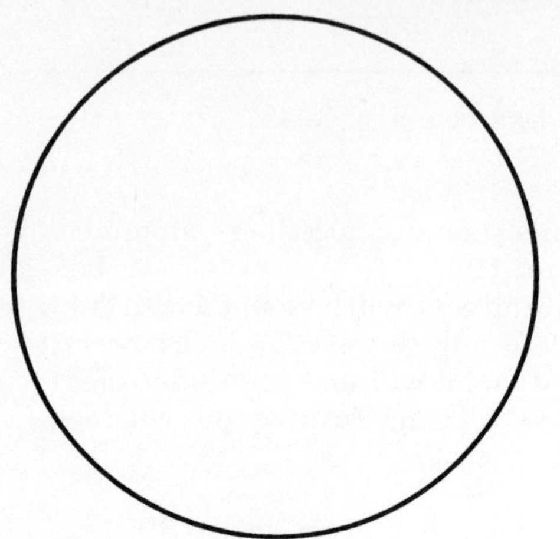

Figure 9–1. Object _____________

Magnification × _____

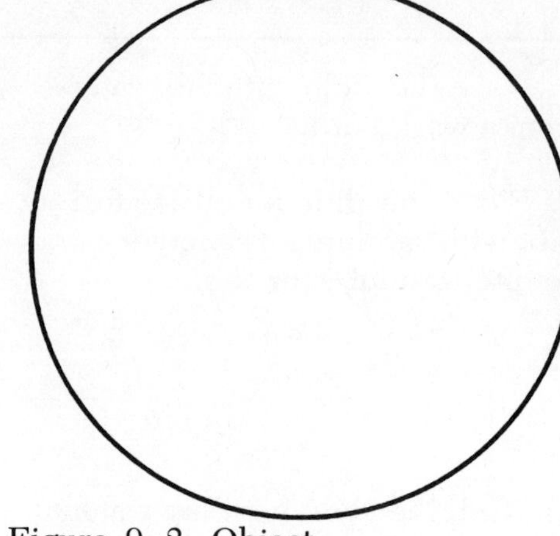

Figure 9–2. Object _____________

Magnification ×_____

Figure 9–3. Object _____________

Magnification ×_____

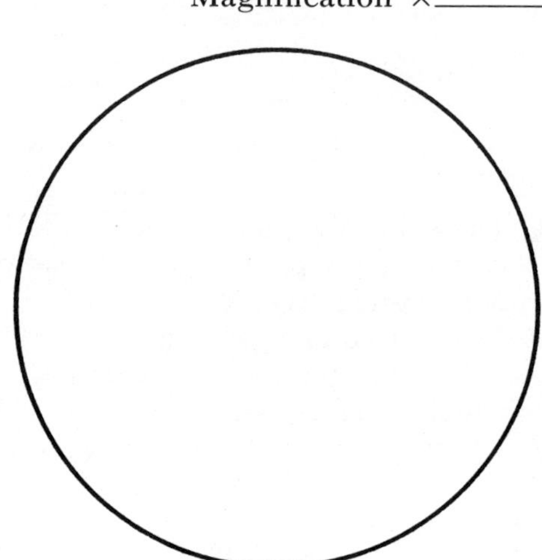

Figure 9–4. Object _____________

Magnification ×_____

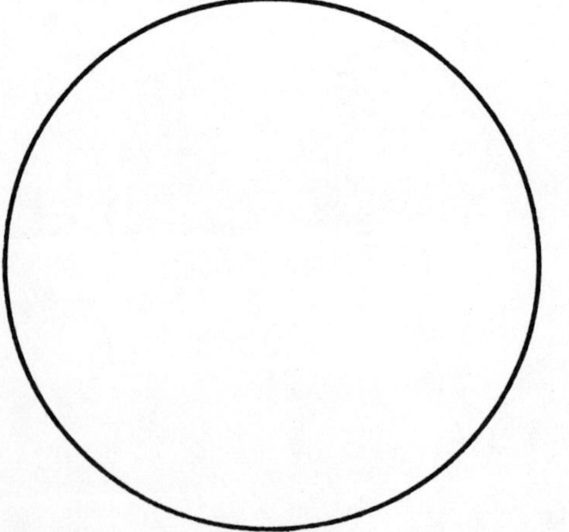

Figure 9–5. Object _____________

Magnification ×_____

Questions:

1. Define:

   a. Primary stain

   b. Mordant

   c. Decolorizing agent

   d. Counterstain

2. The advantage of Gram's stain over simple staining is _________________

   ____.

3. Gram-positive organisms retain the ________________________________

   of _________________________________ and gram-negative organisms are

   colored _________________because of _______________________________.

4. Discuss briefly theories of the Gram stain.

Laboratory Exercise 10

TOPIC: ACID-FAST STAINING

OBJECTIVES:
1. To give the student experience with the technique of acid-fast staining.
2. To acquaint the student with some important acid-fast organisms.
3. To demonstrate a method of differentiating bacteria by means of the acid-fast stain.

EQUIPMENT:
1. 72 hr broth culture of *Enterobacter aerogenes.*
2. 72 hr agar culture (or older if necessary) of *Mycobacterium smegmatis.*
3. Autoclaved sputum from individual who has active tuberculosis.
4. Carbolfuchsin Ziehl-Neelsen stain.
5. Acid alcohol (3 per cent concentrated HCl in 95 per cent alcohol).
6. Methylene blue.
7. Water bath or metal staining pan (or a slide warmer).
8. Filter paper.

Procedure:

KEY STEPS	IMPORTANT POINTS
1. Prepare smears of *Enterobacter aerogenes* and *Mycobacterium smegmatis* as outlined in Exercise 8.	1.1. See Exercise 8.
2. Cover the smears with a piece of filter paper.	2.1. The filter paper prevents crystals of the stain from forming on the smear.
3. Flood the slide with carbolfuchsin (saturate the filter paper and keep it saturated).	3.1. See Exercise 8.
4. Steam by *one* of the following methods for 5 min: a. The flame of the Bunsen burner (*do not boil*). b. On a metal staining pan, with the flame inserted below the slide. c. Over a water bath. d. On a slide warmer.	4.1. Because of the waxy consistency or substance of acid-fast bacteria, the stain must be steamed into the cells. 4.2. The most convenient, inexpensive method for steaming stains on smears is a metal pan with a piece of screen wire across the top covering about half the pan. The slide rests on the screen wire. The burner can easily be inserted below so that the flame will briefly heat the slide. 4.3. If a water bath is used, the water must be kept steaming for the entire staining time. 4.4. It is frequently necessary to replenish the dye at intervals during the staining period. ***Do not let the filter paper get dry.*** 4.5. Some workers prefer not to cover the stain with filter paper. In this case, care must *especially* be taken not to let the smear go dry.

KEY STEPS	**IMPORTANT POINTS**
5. Gently remove the filter paper.	5.1. If not removed gently, the paper may adhere to the smear and remove it from the slide.
6. Wash the dye off with tap water.	6.1. See Exercise 8.
7. Decolorize with acid alcohol, tilting the slide until no more dye comes off (approximately 30 sec). It should be slightly pink.	7.1. There is greater danger of overdecolorization with acid alcohol in this stain than with acetone alcohol in the Gram stain.
8. Flood the slide with methylene blue for 1 min.	8.1. Methylene blue is the counterstain in this procedure.
9. Wash and blot the slide dry. Examine the slide, using the oil immersion lens of the microscope.	9.1. See Exercise 8.
10. Obtain a prepared smear of sputum containing **Mycobacterium tuberculosis** from your instructor. Stain as just directed.	10.1. Sputum containing **M. tuberculosis** is highly infectious and should not be handled by inexperienced people. It is desirable to autoclave this material; this does not affect the stain. 10.2. If the smear is completely dry and well fixed to the slide, it is not infectious. However, it is important to be intelligently cautious and there is no need to touch the smear with your fingers.

Record of Results:

1. Make drawings in color of each of the slides examined under the oil immersion objective. Indicate which organisms were acid-fast and which were not acid-fast.

Questions:

1. By acid-fastness is meant ____

____.

2. Two pathogenic organisms which are acid-fast are _____________________________

and ____.

3. One nonpathogenic organism which is acid-fast is ______________________________.

4. This property of acid-fastness may be due to _______________________

____.

5. The primary stain in this acid-fast staining procedure is _______________

____.

6. The decolorizing agent in this acid-fast staining procedure is _______________

____.

7. The counterstain in this acid-fast staining procedure is _______________

____.

Drawings of Organisms Seen After Acid-fast Staining

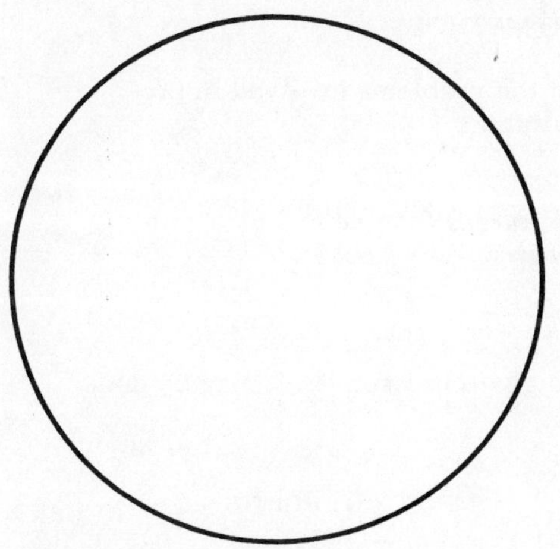

Figure 10–1. Object ______________

Magnification × ______

Figure 10–2. Object ______________

Magnification × ______

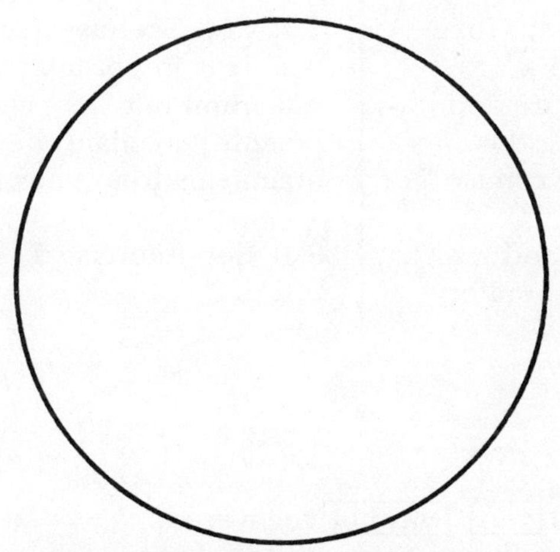

Figure 10–3. Object ______________

Magnification × ______

Laboratory Exercise 11

TOPIC: PURE CULTURE TECHNIQUE (STREAK PLATE METHOD)

OBJECTIVE: 1. To give the student an appreciation of the problems involved in preparing a pure culture from a mixed culture.

EQUIPMENT: 1. Mixed broth culture of *Staphylococcus aureus* (nonpathogenic strain), *Serratia marcescens,* and *Escherichia coli.**
2. Sterile nutrient agar in tube for plating.
3. Sterile Petri dish.

Procedure: (This experiment, based on the techniques given in Exercise 7, may be done at the same time as Experiment 12.)

KEY STEPS	**IMPORTANT POINTS**
1. Pour sterile nutrient agar plates as indicated in Exercise 7.	1.1. See Exercise 7. Pour either from medium in tubes or from an Erlenmeyer flask.
2. After the agar is hard, sterilize the inoculating loop; take a loopful of the mixed culture and streak the agar plate using the method diagrammed in Exercise 7.	2.1. See Exercise 7. 2.2. It is important that you spread the inoculum out very well so that you will be able to isolate the three different organisms from your plates.
3. Label your Petri dish and incubate until the next laboratory period.	3.1. See Exercise 7, Steps 8.1., 8.2., 8.3., 9.1., 9.2.

Results:

1. *Staphylococcus aureus* ⬛was⬛ ⬛was not⬛ recovered.
   How did you determine the recovery of this organism?

2. *Serratia marcescens* ⬛was⬛ ⬛was not⬛ recovered.
   How did you determine the recovery of this organism?

---

*Instead of incubating these organisms together, it is better to grow them separately and mix the cultures just before use by adding 1 ml of each culture to a sterile tube. *S. marcescens* tends to overgrow the other two organisms if they are grown together in a mixed culture. *Micrococcus luteus (Sarcina lutea),* which mutates easily to the white variety, may also be used instead of *S. marcescens.* If *Micrococcus* is used, the student should see previously prepared plates of *Staphylococcus aureus* and *Micrococcus luteus (Sarcina lutea)* to appreciate the differences in pigmentation produced.

3. ***Escherichia coli*** ☐ was ☐ was not recovered.
   How did you determine the recovery of this organism?

Record of Observations:

1. Record observations made after the incubation period. Did the plate contain isolated colonies of the three original organisms?

Questions:

1. The value of this procedure in isolating pure cultures from a mixed culture is

   ____

   ____.

2. Organisms in the environment are usually found in _______________________

   ____ ☐ pure culture ☐ mixed culture

3. a. When you send nose, throat or stool specimens to the laboratory for examination, are these mixed or pure cultures?

   b. In order to determine if there are pathogenic organisms in these specimens, what does the laboratory technician have to do?

Laboratory Exercise 12

TOPIC: PURE CULTURE TECHNIQUE (POUR PLATE METHOD)

OBJECTIVE: 1. To demonstrate to the student an additional method of preparing pure cultures from mixed cultures.

EQUIPMENT: 1. Mixed broth culture of *Staphylococcus aureus* (nonpathogenic stain), *Serratia marcescens,* and *Escherichia coli.**
2. Sterile nutrient agar in tubes for plating.
3. Sterile Petri dish.

Procedure: (Students should have enough information to fill in some of the important points for themselves.)

KEY STEPS	IMPORTANT POINTS
1. Heat the tube containing the sterile nutrient agar in a water bath or beaker of water until the agar is liquefied. Cool to 45-50 C.	1.1. See Exercise 7, Steps 1.1., 2.1., 2.2.
2. With a sterile inoculating loop, take a loopful of the mixed culture and put it in the tube of melted and slightly cooled agar. You may also use a sterile pipette for a drop inoculation.	2.1. The temperature of the agar must not be above 50 C because _______________________________. 2.2. The temperature of the agar must not be below 40 C because _______________________________.
3. Rotate the tube containing the liquid nutrient agar quickly between the palms of your hands, flame briefly and pour the agar immediately into a sterile Petri dish. Rotate the agar gently on the bottom of the dish.	3.1. The inoculating tube containing the nutrient agar is rotated because _______________________________. 3.2. It is important to work quickly at this point because _______________________________.
4. Allow the nutrient agar to harden; label the Petri dish and incubate as described in Exercise 7.	4.1. It is easier to pick colonies from a smooth surface than one that is rough from agitation during hardening. 4.2. See Exercise 7, Steps 8.1., 8.2., 8.3., 9.1., 9.2.

---

*See footnote for Exercise 11, page 60.

Results:

1. Record all results after the incubation period. Compare with the results of Exercise 11.

   a. ***Staphylococcus aureus*** was was not recovered. How did you determine the recovery of this organism?

   b. ***Serratia marcescens*** was was not recovered.
   How did you determine the recovery of this organism?

   c. ***Escherichia coli*** was was not recovered.
   How did you determine the recovery of this organism?

Note: This experiment requires that nutrient agar be inoculated prior to pouring the plates. Another, very useful technique involves dilutions of the samples; this will be done in a later experiment. In this technique, aliquots of samples with the organisms in them are pipetted to sterile Petri plates; then the liquid, cooled (40–50 C) nutrient agar is poured over the samples. The Petri dishes are gently rotated to mix the bacteria and the medium. See Experiment 7, Step 4.2.

Questions:

1. What is the purpose of "plating-out" cultures?

2. Why is it difficult, or impossible, to positively identify microorganisms in a mixed culture?

3. What are the advantages of pure cultures?

4. Is the pour plate or the streak plate method better for isolating organisms from a mixed culture? Why?

5. The appearance of colonies of some organisms in a pour plate differs from that of the same organisms on a streak plate. Why?

6. What happens to the organisms that are below the surface of the medium in the plates?

Laboratory Exercise 13

TOPIC: ORGANISMS IN THE ENVIRONMENT

OBJECTIVE: 1. To give the student an appreciation of the widespread distribution of microorganisms in the environment.

EQUIPMENT: 1. Tubes of sterile nutrient agar for plating.
2. Sterile Petri dishes.
3. Sterile cotton applicators (dry and moist).*

Procedure:

KEY STEPS	IMPORTANT POINTS
1. Prepare sterile nutrient agar plates as described in Exercise 7; Step 4.2 is preferred.	1.1. See Exercise 7.
2. Select some object in the environment to culture.	2.1. In consultation with your instructor, select some object or substance that you would like to investigate from the viewpoint of microbiology. Try to have as much variety in the class as possible by having students culture different objects (see suggestions listed below).
3. Streak the agar plates and label as indicated in Exercise 7, Steps 7 and 8.	3.1. See Exercise 7.
4. Incubate as stated in Exercise 7, Step 9.	4.1. See Exercise 7.

Suggestions of Objects to Culture:

1. *Air*
   a. Expose the nutrient agar plate to air for 5 min by removing the cover. Keep the cover with the inside down for the exposure period.
   b. Repeat the same exposure at various levels of the room, i.e., on top of a tall cabinet, on the laboratory desk, on the floor.
2. *Hair*
   a. Remove a hair from your scalp with a previously flamed forceps and drop it on sterile nutrient agar in a Petri dish.
3. *Fingers*
   a. Streak the fingers of one hand across the surface of the agar. Be careful not to break the nutrient agar.

---

*See footnote for Exercise 7, page 39.

4. ***Dry Objects or Surfaces*** (coins, shower floors, toilet seats, bottom of shoe, finger-nails, etc.)
   a. With a sterile moist cotton applicator, swab an area selected for culture.
   b. Streak a sterile nutrient agar plate with this contaminated applicator.
5. ***Dusting***
   a. Hold a sterile nutrient agar plate just below a window sill while another student dusts half of the window sill with a dry duster.
   b. After a few minutes repeat 5a, using a second sterile agar plate and a damp duster on the second half of the same window sill.
6. ***Sweeping***
   a. Place a sterile nutrient agar plate on a rug.
   b. Sweep the rug with a broom near the plate.
   c. After 5 min repeat with a second agar plate, using a vacuum sweeper instead of a broom. (This may not show too much difference unless a rug is selected which is not extremely dusty.)

Record of Results:

1. Record the growth obtained on your plates and those of other students in the laboratory section.
2. Make a record of the numbers and kinds of colonies found on these plates.

GROWTH OF COLONIES FROM THE ENVIRONMENT ON NUTRIENT AGAR PLATES

Source of Culture	Temperature of Incubation	Amount of Growth	Shape of Colonies	Color	Consistency of Colonies	Drawings of Typical Colonies*

*See page 201 in the appendix.

Questions:

1. Most organisms in the environment are _______________________
   (pathogenic, nonpathogenic).

2. Damp dusting is preferred to dry dusting because _______________

   ____.

3. Cleaning rugs with a vacuum sweeper is preferred to sweeping with a broom be-

   cause ____

   ____.

4. Fingers should be kept away from your face and mouth except while eating because

   ____

   ____.

5. Hair should be well controlled when working with patients because _________

   ____

   ____.

6. Hands should be washed thoroughly before serving patients' trays and before eating

   because ____

   ____

   ____.

7. The number and species of organisms in the air may vary at different levels because

   ____

   ____

   ____.

Laboratory Exercise 14

TOPIC: PROTEIN HYDROLYSIS

OBJECTIVES: 1. To show the action of microbial enzymes produced by some bacteria.
2. To give a clearer understanding of enzymes which act on some proteins.

EQUIPMENT: 1. 24 hr broth culture of *Bacillus subtilis.*
2. 24 hr broth culture of *Enterobacter liquefaciens* or *Serratia marcescens.*
3. 24 hr broth culture of *Enterobacter cloacae.*
4. 24 hr broth culture of *Escherichia coli.*
5. Five tubes of sterile nutrient gelatin (8 g nutrient broth, 100 g gelatin,* 1 liter distilled water).

Procedure:

KEY STEPS	IMPORTANT POINTS
1. Place the tubes of nutrient gelatin in ice water, or in a refrigerator.	1.1. Gelatin is chilled because _________ _________.
2. Label each tube carefully with the name of one organism, the medium, the date and your initials.	2.1. Accurate labeling is important because _________ _________.
3. Inoculate by stabbing the wire into the gelatin without allowing the holder of the needle to touch the surface of the gelatin. Use a different culture for each of the three tubes and save one tube for the uninoculated control.	3.1. This type of inoculation produces a stab culture. 3.2. In a stab culture some organisms grow the entire length of the stab and others grow only on the surface. Explain why.
4. Incubate as described in Exercise 7.	4.1. See Exercise 7. (25 C may be preferable for some cultures.)
5. At the next laboratory period place all tubes, including the control, in a beaker of ice-cold water, or for 30 min in the refrigerator.	5.1. The tubes are chilled because _________ _________. 5.2. The purpose of the control tube is _________ _________. 5.3. Note that gelatin liquefaction for the same organism in the same tube may be checked after 24 hr, 48 hr, 72 hr, and so on, by putting the tubes back in the incubator after the exposure to cold temperature. Organisms may liquefy gelatin in 72 hr but not in 48 hr, and so forth.

---

*Difco prefers 12% gelatin.

Record of Obervations:

1. After sufficient time has elapsed to allow for solidification of the gelatin in the uninoculated control tube, note if liquefaction has occurred in any of the tubes. (Thirty minutes should be enough time to show if the gelatin remains liquid in the cold.) Check after 1 day's incubation, after 2 days' incubation, and after 3 days' incubation of the gelatin.
2. Note the type of growth that has occurred in the gelatin.

Culture	Incubation Time at 37C	Liquefaction	Type of Growth
Bacillus subtilis	24 hr		
	48 hr		
	72 hr		
*Enterobacter liquefaciens** or *Serratia marcescens*	24 hr		
	48 hr		
	72 hr		
Escherichia coli	24 hr		
	48 hr		
	72 hr		
Enterobacter cloacae	24 hr		
	48 hr		
	72 hr		
Uninoculated control	72 hr		

Enterobacter liquefaciens* may be a nonpigmented species of **Serratia. It is no longer recognized as a species of **Enterobacter.** Refer to Bergey's Manual of Determinative Bacteriology, Eighth Edition, 1974, pages 292 and 324.

Questions:

1. The disadvantages for isolating pure cultures by using gelatin media are _____

   _______________________________ and ____________________________.

2. The enzyme which hydrolyzes gelatin is called _________________________.

3. Three other enzymes which attack protein are _________________________,

   _______________________________ and ____________________________.

4. Four products of enzyme digestion of proteins are _________________________,

   ___________________, ___________________ and ________________________.

Laboratory Exercise 15

TOPIC: CARBOHYDRATE DIGESTION OR HYDROLYSIS—FERMENTATION

OBJECTIVES: 1. To study the action of some bacteria on carbohydrates.
2. To give a better understanding of enzyme action.
3. To study a very useful differential medium, TSI.

EQUIPMENT: 1. 24 hr broth culture of *Pseudomonas fluorescens.*
2. 24 hr broth culture of *Escherichia coli.*
3. 24 hr broth culture of *Enterobacter aerogenes.*
4. 24 hr broth culture of *Proteus vulgaris.*
5. Five Durham tubes of glucose broth with phenol red indicator.*
6. Five Durham tubes of sucrose broth with bromcresol purple indicator.
7. Five Durham tubes of lactose broth with phenol red indicator.
8. Five slants of TSI Agar (Triple Sugar Iron Agar, available from BBL).

Procedure:

KEY STEPS	IMPORTANT POINTS
1. Inoculate a different organism into each of three tubes of glucose broth. Repeat with lactose and sucrose broth. Keep one tube of each kind of broth for an uninoculated control.	1.1. You used three different organisms and three different sugar broths because ________ ________________________________ ______________________________. 1.2. The purposes of the control tubes of broth are ______________________ _____________________________.
2. Inoculate each culture into each of four tubes of TSI agar by stabbing with a straight needle into the slant to the butt of the tube, pull up and streak.	2.1. Note the meanings of the reactions that may be observed on this "one" differential medium as indicated on the list shown below.
3. Incubate as previously described.	3.1. See Exercise 7.

LIST OF RANGES OF pH FOR SOME INDICATORS

		Acidic—Basic
Phenol red (0.02% recommended)	pH 6.8–8.4	color range, yellow-red
Bromcresol purple (0.04% recommended)	pH 5.2–6.8	color range, yellow-purple
Bromthymol blue (0.04% recommended)	pH 6.0–7.6	color range, yellow-blue

To make up the indicators use 0.01 N NaOH (28.2 ml for phenol red, 18.5 ml for bromcresol purple, and 16.0 ml for bromthymol blue) with 0.1 g of the indicator dye, and dilute to 250 ml with distilled water for the 0.04% solutions (to 125 ml for phenol red). (Reference: Difco Manual, 9th ed., page 295.)

---

*Phenol Red Broth Base is commercially available from Difco Laboratories and requires only the addition of a carbohydrate, such as glucose, sucrose, lactose, maltose, xylose, and so forth.

REACTIONS OBSERVED ON TSI AGAR*

Reaction Observed†	Type of Fermentation
Acid butt (yellow), alkaline slant (red)	Glucose fermented
Acid throughout medium, butt and slant yellow	Lactose or sucrose or both fermented
Gas bubbles in butt, medium may split	Aerogenic culture
Blackening of butt	Hydrogen sulfide produced
Alkaline slant and butt (medium entirely red)	None of the three sugars fermented

*From Bailey and Scott: Diagnostic Microbiology, 1970, St. Louis, C. V. Mosby Co.
†Note that the reactions observed are not exclusive (H_2S can be produced, also bubbles, and so forth).

INTERPRETATION OF REACTIONS ON TSI AGAR*

Reaction	Carbohydrates fermented	Possible organisms
Acid butt Acid slant Gas in butt No H_2S	Glucose with acid and gas Lactose and/or sucrose with acid and gas	*Escherichia* *Klebsiella* or *Enterobacter* *Proteus* Intermediate coliforms
Acid butt Alkaline slant Gas in butt H_2S	Glucose with acid and gas Lactose and sucrose not fermented	*Salmonella* *Proteus* *Salmonella arizonae* (certain strains) *Citrobacter* (certain types) *Edwardsiella*
Acid butt Alkaline slant No gas in butt No H_2S	Glucose with acid only Lactose and sucrose not fermented	*Salmonella*† *Shigella* *Proteus* *Serratia*
Acid butt Acid slant Gas in butt H_2S produced	Glucose with acid and gas Lactose and/or sucrose with acid and gas	*Salmonella arizonae* *Citrobacter*
Alkaline or neutral butt Alkaline slant No H_2S	None	*Alcaligenes*‡ *Pseudomonas*‡ *Herellea*‡

*From Bailey and Scott: Diagnostic Microbiology, 1970, St. Louis, C. V. Mosby Co.
†*Salmonella typhi* produces a small amount of H_2S but seldom gas.
‡Included here because colonies of these may be confused frequently with lactose-negative members of Enterobacteriaceae and may be selected from isolation plates.

Questions:

1. Four enzymes which act on carbohydrates are _______________________,

   _______________________, _______________________ and _______________________.

2. Two gases which are formed in breaking down carbohydrates are _______________________

   _______________________and _______________________.

3. Four other products of carbohydrate decomposition are _______________________,

   _______________________, _______________________and _______________________.

4. State how the organisms used in this exercise may be differentiated by their
   carbohydrate metabolism.

5. What advantages can you see in using TSI agar over the three carbohydrate fermentation media? _______________________

   _______________________.

Record of Results:
1. Note the changes of color of the media.
2. Note the presence or absence of gas in the Durham tubes.
3. Note the reactions on TSI agar.

RESULTS OF ACTION OF BACTERIA ON CARBOHYDRATES

Culture	Glucose		Sucrose		Lactose		TSI agar			
	Acid	Gas	Acid	Gas	Acid	Gas	Slant Acid	Butt Acid	Butt Gas	H₂S
Uninoculated control										
Pseudomonas fluorescens										
Escherichia coli										
Enterobacter aerogenes										
Proteus vulgaris										

Incubation time, 48 hr at 37 C.
Acid is yellow on TSI.
Alkaline is red on TSI.

Laboratory Exercise 16

TOPIC: MORPHOLOGY AND REPRODUCTION OF RICKETTSIAS AND VIRUSES

OBJECTIVE: 1. To help the students to understand ultramicroscopic forms of microorganisms, i.e., rickettsias and viruses (including bacteriophage).
2. To show how bacteriophage may be obtained and reproduced.

EQUIPMENT: 1. 2 × 2 or 3¼ × 4 projection slides of electron micrographs of rickettsias and viruses (see Appendix for possible sources).
2. Suitable projector and screen.
3. 250 ml nutrient broth in a 3 liter flask. Sterility is not required.
4. Feces, 10 to 20 g emulsified in water, or an equally rich soil sample, or polluted river sample.*
5. Test organisms (potential hosts) like **Escherichia, Pseudomonas,** or **Salmonella** (if your instructor is brave) in a broth culture.
6. Some nutrient agar Petri plates seeded with the test organisms (see Item 5), incubated 24 hr.
7. A sterile bacterial filter.
8. Some large filter paper and a funnel.

KEY STEPS	IMPORTANT POINTS
1. The instructor will show slides of rickettsias and viruses.	1.1. Are rickettsias and viruses alike or different in structure? Explain. 1.2. Why are rickettsias important to the health professions? 1.3. Why are viruses important to the health professions?
2. This may be a demonstration or it can be done in groups. Add the feces sample to the 250 ml nutrient broth, shake well and add 1 ml of the test organism. This is called **enriching** the phage.	2.1. This isolation of a phage may be extended over several laboratory periods, or preparations may be made prior to this exercise. 2.2. The student should keep in mind that there is only a certain amount of chance that a specific phage for a specific phage-host (bacteria) may be isolated from a certain sample of feces. What are your chances?
3. Incubate for 24 hr, shaking occasionally. Keep overnight in a refrigerator, then filter the supernatant through several layers of nonsterile filter paper.	3.1. Why is sterility not required here; at least for your purposes?

*If your instructor obtains specific phage for Item 4 commercially and the specific phage-host for Item 5 the chances that this experiment will work are greatly increased.

KEY STEPS	**IMPORTANT POINTS**
4. Filter the filtrate through a sterile bacterial filter.	4.1. A sterile bacterial filter may be an asbestos pad filter, Zeitz filter; a membrane filter like the Millipore or the Falcon; sintered glass filters; Micro-filters, syringe fitted. How many of these filters have you seen in the laboratory or in pictures? 4.2. What is the purpose of these filters?
5. Place loopful amounts of the filtrate on the bacterial lawn of the seeded Petri plates (Equipment 6.). Incubate overnight.	5.1. One problem in bacteriophage studies is that unless the relative concentrations of the phage and its host are just right you may not see plaques. Also, the time required for the formation of plaques is very important; so are phage resistant mutants that may arise. They are called lysogenic strains.
6. If phage is present it should form plaques on the bacterial lawn — these holes in the growth are due to lysis of the bacteria by the bacteriophage.	6.1. If you wish you may scrape out single plaques, enrich, dilute and purify the phage, thus building up a phage stock. Note that this is time consuming and is not required here.

Record of Results:
1. Draw representatives of rickettsias and viruses, including bacteriophage. Your sources are your textbook, other books, or illustrations of electron micrographs you are shown in the laboratory. Do not expect to see simple viruses with your microscope! Why?
2. Record any likenesses and differences between rickettsias and viruses.
3. What does the plate with bacteriophage plaques look like?

Drawings of Rickettsias and Viruses

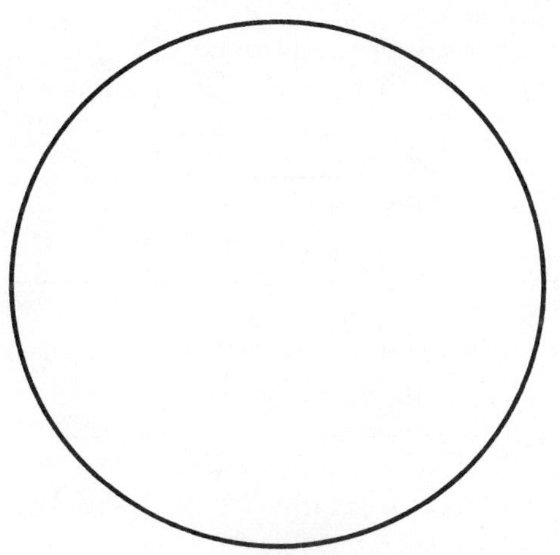

Figure 16–1. Object ________________

Magnification × ______

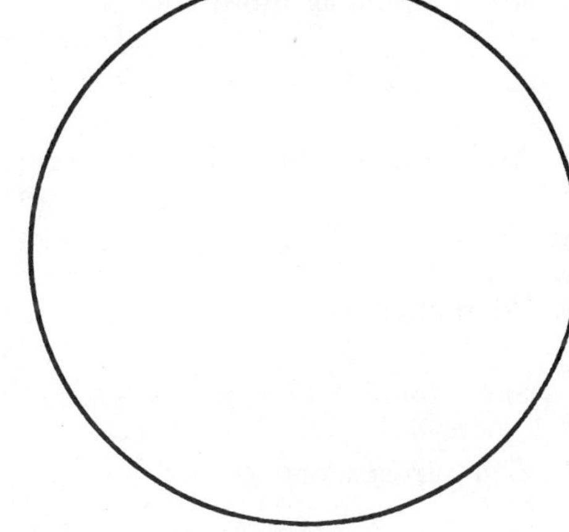

Figure 16–2. Object ________________

Magnification × ______

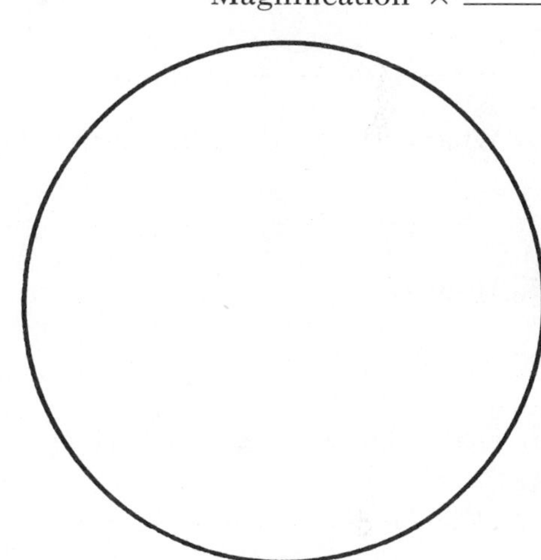

Figure 16–3. Object ________________

Magnification × ______

Figure 16–4. Object ________________

Magnification × ______

Figures 16–1 to 16–4 are drawings of illustrations shown in the laboratory.

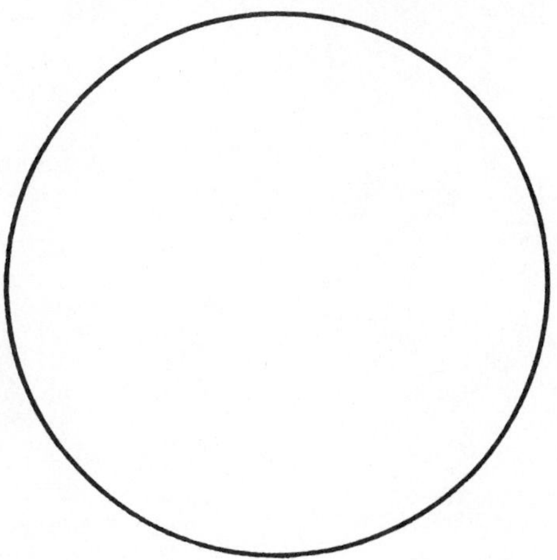

Figure 16–5. Object: Petri plate
showing plaques of bacteriophage. Magnification about half
size, host organism used

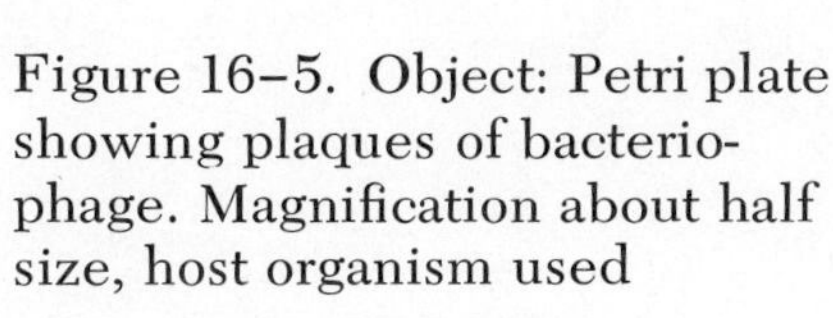

Questions:

1. Are rickettsias more like microscopic plants or microscopic animals? _________

   ____

2. Are viruses more like microscopic plants or microscopic animals?_____________

   ____

3. What characteristics of some viruses indicate that this group of microorganisms has

   some inanimate features?____

4. Can viruses and rickettsias live in cultures without living cells in the media? _

   ____

5. What is the relationship of size of rickettsias to common bacteria?_____________

   ____

6. What is the relationship of the size of viruses to common bacteria? ____________

   ____

7. How are bacteria affected by bacteriophage? _________________________________

   ____

8. Do we know more about bacteriophage than about other viruses? If your answer is

   yes, explain.____

   ____

   ____

Unit Two

PHYSICAL AND CHEMICAL AGENTS AS METHODS OF INHIBITING AND/OR KILLING BACTERIA

Each day workers in the health fields must make decisions about inhibition, destruction and removal of microorganisms which may come from any patient in any kind of hospital or public health nursing situation. For example, fresh linen is not sterile but is clean and in almost all cases free from pathogenic microorganisms. However, linen removed from a patient's bed is contaminated with any microorganism the patient harbors. Therefore, this linen should be folded neatly and placed on a cart, or in a hamper, in the patient's unit (not thrown in an unsightly mess on the floor) and carried to the linen chute or receptacle, being careful not to hold the linen against one's own clothing, or especially, one's own body or face. Linen from a patient with a known communicable disease should be placed in a separate bag, carefully labeled with a red tag for the protection of laundry personnel and handled by the laundry in such a way as to prevent any spread of microorganisms.

In addition, there are many pieces of equipment used daily in the care of patients that become contaminated during their use and must be disinfected or sterilized before reuse. The exercises in this unit are designed to show the contamination of some of these articles of equipment and some of the methods of disinfection or sterilization. Hospital personnel must be aware of the fact that in the practice of their professions they never, never encounter "naked" organisms. Rather, they are dealing with microorganisms protected by some form of protein found in blood, secretions and excretions. This means that time factors and dilutions of chemicals studied only on naked organisms are not reliable for hospital practice. More testing under conditions of actual use needs to be done.

It is essential to learn more about different characteristics of pathogenic microorganisms and to recognize the need for special procedures of disinfection or sterilization in caring for patients with known communicable diseases.

Also, because hospital personnel's hands are in direct contact with so many items in every patient's unit, the author feels that too little attention is being paid by the practitioners of the health professions to hand washing. It is possible that newer methods of adequately cleaning hands can be developed which would be less time consuming than traditional methods of hand washing. However, at present, adequate hand washing with plenty of soap and water and conscientious attention to cleansing all parts of the hand is the only known method of removing recent contaminants. The rigorous scrubbing of hands in the operating room followed by chemical disinfection and donning of sterile gloves is essential to prevent the transfer of normal skin inhabitants to tissue exposed by surgical incisions.

The situations just described are only a few of the many uses of the knowledge of inhibition and destruction of microorganisms. The author recommends that each beginning student keep a record of the incidents and situations that require this knowledge and indicate what specific method of inhibition, destruction or removal of microorganisms was used in each.

Laboratory Exercise 17

TOPIC: EFFECT OF DRYING ON MICROORGANISMS

OBJECTIVES: 1. To show the effect of drying on bacteria.
2. To show the practical application of this in the patient's care and in the preservation of food.

EQUIPMENT: 1. 5 day old broth culture of *Bacillus subtilis.*
2. 48 hr broth culture of *Serratia marcescens.*
3. 48 hr broth culture of *Escherichia coli.*
4. Two sterile test tubes.
5. Sterile nutrient broth.
6. One sterile 10 ml pipette.
7. Three sterile 1 ml pipettes.

Procedure:

KEY STEPS	IMPORTANT POINTS
1. Using a sterile 1 ml pipette, place a drop of a **B. subtilis** culture in the bottom of a sterile test tube. Use good aseptic technique. Repeat, placing a drop of either **S. marcescens** or **E. coli** cultures in a second sterile test tube.	1.1. A drop of culture in the tube of medium would produce a good subculture of the original organism. 1.2. Are moisture and food essential to growth? Why? 1.3. Pipettes are often used for drop-inoculations to sterile tubes or media.
2. Label and place in your desk for 1 week.	2.1. Why should you leave these tubes for 1 week?
3. At the end of 1 week, put 3 ml of sterile nutrient broth in each tube. Use a sterile pipette to transfer the broth to the tube.	3.1. Why do you need to add broth to the tubes? 3.2. Why must you use a sterile pipette to transfer the broth to the tubes?
4. Put the tubes in your desk for 1 week.	4.1. Why do these tubes need to be incubated? 5.1. Practice of proper pipetting techniques is essential for good laboratory work.

Record of Observations:

1. Note the growth in each tube and record. Describe the type of growth observed for each organism.

Questions:

1. **Bacillus subtilis** $\boxed{\text{showed}}$ $\boxed{\text{did not show}}$ growth because ___________

____.

2. *Serratia marcescens* | showed | | did not show | growth because ___________________

____.

3. *Escherichia coli* | showed | | did not show | growth because ___________________

____.

4. State the application of this experiment to hospital care.

5. State how these principles have been used in food preservation.

6. What are the advantages of pipetting a drop versus inoculating with a loop needle?

1. Before pipetting, the sterile pipette can containing the sterile pipettes is opened as shown and the mouthpieces of the pipettes are exposed to the air. After pipetting each pipette is deposited in the jar containing 5% Lysol, to be washed at a later time.

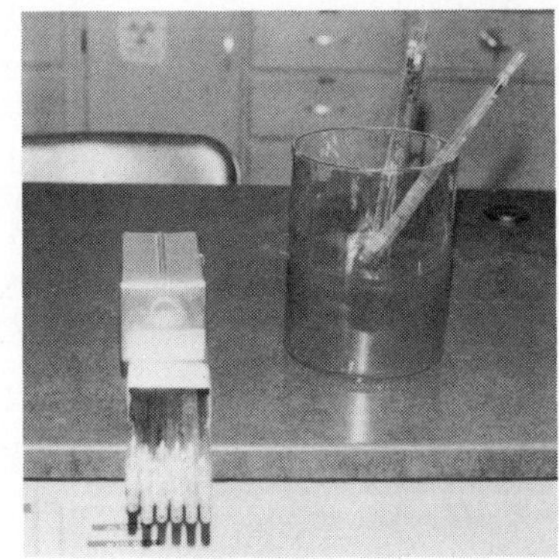

2. There is only one right way to pick up a sterile pipette. It is shown in this figure. The forefinger, never the thumb, is placed over the opening. The pipette must never touch any surface, other than the inside of the flask or tube from where the fluid is to be pipetted into another flask, tube or plate and the fluid itself. If an outside (contaminated) surface is accidentally touched, the pipette is immediately discarded into the Lysol jar.

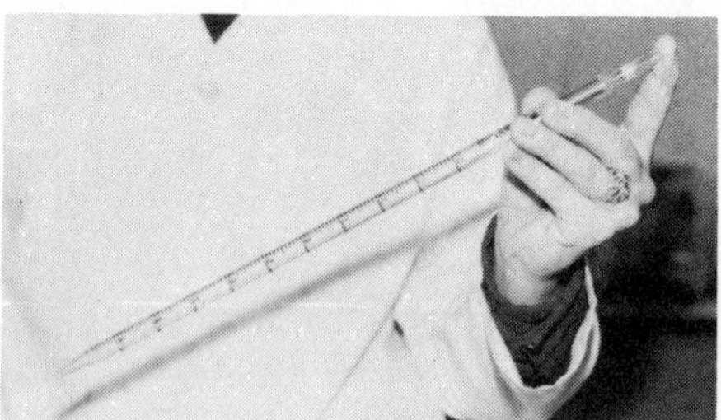

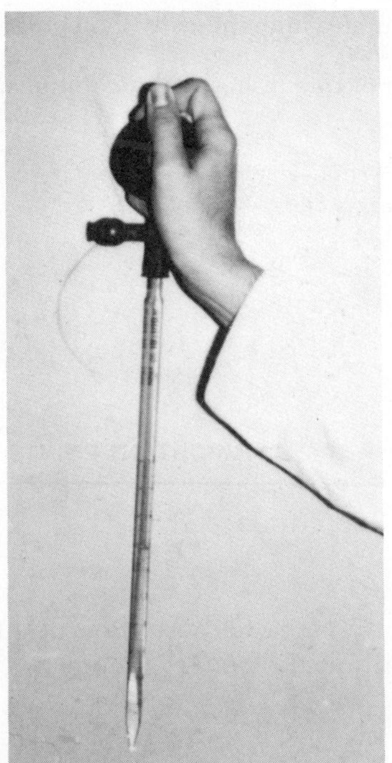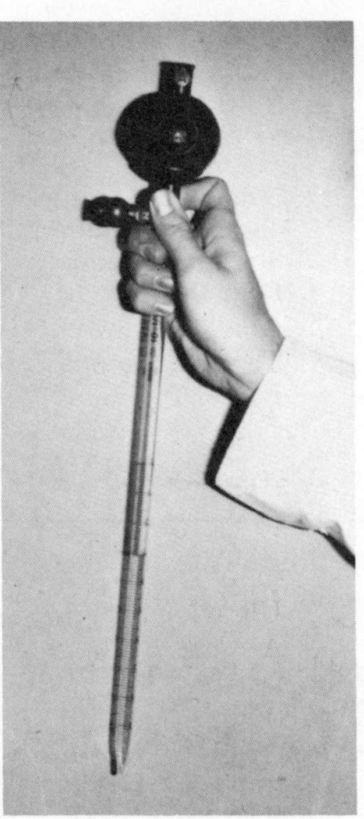

This propipette consists of a bulb which is attachable to any size pipette by pressing valve A and compressing the bulb in the fist (see *A*). Draw the liquid up by pressing valve S on stem. To release liquid press valve E on side of stem (see *B*).

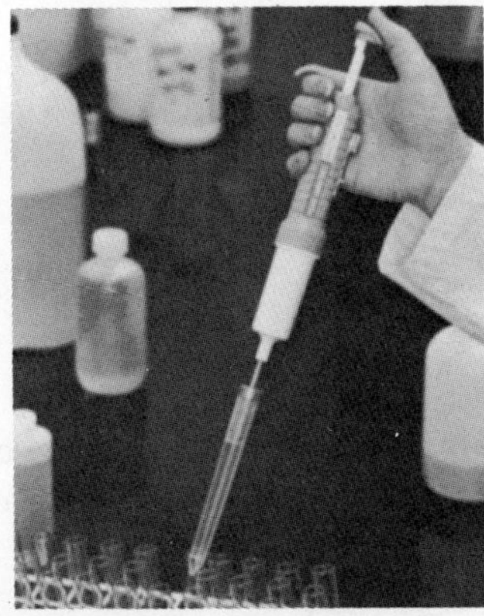

This pipette filler represents one of several models of pipetting devices available commercially. All are somewhat different. Some have precalibrated disposable tips that are usually highly accurate. They can be used for sterile techniques.

Laboratory Exercise 18

TOPIC: INHIBITING ACTION OF SUNLIGHT ON MICROORGANISMS

OBJECTIVES: 1. To demonstrate the action of sunlight, a high intensity light bulb or ultra-violet light on bacteria.
2. To show the practical application of this in hospital techniques.

MATERIALS: 1. 5 day broth culture of *Bacillus subtilis.*
2. 48 hr broth culture of *Serratia marcescens.*
3. Sterile nutrient agar.
4. Four sterile Petri dishes.
5. Ultraviolet lamp.
6. A strong light source or lamp.

Procedure:

KEY STEPS	IMPORTANT POINTS
1. Prepare sterile nutrient agar plates as described in Exercise 7.	1.1. See Exercise 7.
2. After the agar has hardened, turn each Petri dish over and divide the bottom of it in two equal halves, using a wax marking pencil.	2.1. Why is it inadvisable to divide the dishes in half on the cover?
3. Streak one half of each agar plate with **S. *marcescens.***	3.1. Be careful not to cross the line you have made.
4. Streak the second half of each agar plate with **B. *subtilis.***	4.1. See Step 3.1.
5. Expose one Petri dish to the rays of an ultraviolet lamp for 10 min, leaving the cover on. Repeat with the second dish, leaving the cover off.	5.1. Place the Petri dish 15 to 20 inches from the light. 5.2. Would you expect to see differences between these two plates? Why?
6. Expose one Petri dish to the bright sunlight for 10 min, with the cover off.	6.1. How far did this light travel to reach your plate?
7. Expose one Petri dish to a high intensity light bulb for 10 min, leaving the cover off.	7.1. What are the similarities between this light, sunlight, and ultraviolet light? 7.2. Does the heat of the bulb influence the result of your experiment?
8. Keep the fourth plate for a control.	8.1. What are the functions of this control?
9. Label and incubate all Petri dishes.	9.1. How long do you need to incubate these Petri dishes?

Record of Observations:

1. Record the amount and the kind of growth on all plates.*

Nutrient Agar Plates	Growth of *B. subtilis*	Growth of *S. marcescens*
Exposed to ultraviolet light with the cover on		
Exposed to ultraviolet light with the cover off		
Exposed to sunlight		
Exposed to a bright light bulb		
Untreated control		

*Incubated at 25 C for 24 hr.

2. State your conclusions about the effectiveness of the following:

   a. ultraviolet rays

   b. sunlight

   c. high intensity artificial white light

3. List also some experimental factors which occur in this exercise but would not necessarily be present in a practical situation.

Questions:

1. Two situations where ultraviolet lights might be used in a hospital are:

   a.

   b.

2. Ultraviolet rays act on bacterial cells by _______________________

____.

3. State some advantages and disadvantages of this method respective to inhibition and destruction of microorganisms.

4. Sunlight has | favorable | | unfavorable | | no | effects on **B. subtilis** because **B. subtilis**

____.

5. Sunlight has | favorable | | unfavorable | | no | effects on **S. marcescens** because **S.**

marcescens ____

____.

6. The effects of sunlight, if any, are due to _______________________.

7. The effects of the high intensity artificial light (bulb) are due to ___________

____.

Laboratory Exercise 19

TOPIC: EFFECTS OF COLD ON MICROORGANISMS

OBJECTIVES: 1. To show the effect of cold on bacteria.
2. To show the relation between this and the preservation and the storage of food.

EQUIPMENT: 1. 48 hr broth culture of *Bacillus subtilis.*
2. 48 hr broth culture of *Serratia marcescens.*
3. 48 hr broth culture of *Staphylococcus aureus* (nonpathogenic strain).
4. Nine tubes of nutrient broth.

Procedure:

KEY STEPS	IMPORTANT POINTS
1. Inoculate three tubes of nutrient broth with *B. subtilis.* Repeat for *S. marcescens* and for *S. aureus.*	1.1. What sterile technique would you use?
2. Place one tube of each organism in the refrigerator for 1 week, one tube of each organism in the deepfreeze and keep one tube of each organism in your desk for 1 week.	2.1. What is the purpose of these multiple tubes for each organism?
3. After 1 week of refrigeration, make your observation on these tubes and incubate them a second week in your desk.	3.1. Why should you incubate the refrigerated and the frozen tubes in your desk for a second week?

Record of Observations:

1. Record the amount and the kind of growth of each organism incubated in the refrigerator.
2. What happened to the organisms in the deepfreeze?
3. Record the amount and kind of growth of each organism incubated in your desk.
4. Again record after following Step 3 (after incubation for 1 week at room temperature).

GROWTH OF MICROORGANISMS
BEFORE AND AFTER THE SECOND WEEK INCUBATION IN THE DESK

Incubation	*Bacillus subtilis*	*Serratia marcescens*	*Staphylococcus aureus*
Incubated in Your Desk for 1 Week			
Incubated in Your Desk for 2 Weeks			
After 1 Week in the Refrigerator			
After 1 Week in Your Desk, Following Refrigeration			
1 Week in the Deepfreeze			
After 1 Week in Your Desk, Following 1 Week in the Deepfreeze			

Questions:

1. What was the effect of refrigeration on the growth of the microorganisms?

2. In using cold storage or frozen foods, the following precautions must be taken:

    a.

    b.

    c.

3. Practical applications of this experiment in the preservation and storage of food are:

    a.

    b.

    c.

Laboratory Exercise 20

TOPIC: EFFECTS OF DRY HEAT ON MICROORGANISMS

OBJECTIVES:
1. To show the effect of dry heat on bacteria.
2. To show the relation of heat, as a physical agent of destruction of bacteria, to sterile technique.

EQUIPMENT:
1. 5 day broth culture of *Bacillus subtilis.*
2. 5 day broth culture of *Mycobacterium smegmatis.*
3. Two ½ cm sterile gauze squares moistened with a culture of *B. subtilis* in a Petri dish, after 24 hr incubation at 25 C.
4. Two ½ cm sterile gauze squares moistened with *Staphylococcus aureus* (non-pathogenic strain) in a Petri dish, after 24 hr incubation at 37 C.
5. Forceps.
6. Two 5 cm sterile gauze squares in 2 Petri dishes.
7. Sterile nutrient broth in test tubes.
8. Muslin dressing covers or heavy brown paper.
9. Sterile nutrient agar in a flask.
10. Three sterile Petri dishes.

Procedure:

KEY STEPS	IMPORTANT POINTS
A. *Dry Heat-Incineration:*	
1. Prepare three sterile nutrient agar plates.	
2. Divide one plate in half with a wax pencil mark on the bottom.	2.1. See Exercise 18.
3. Using the inoculating loop, streak one complete plate with a loopful of a culture of *B. subtilis.* Flame the inoculating loop. Obtain a second loopful of the culture of *B. subtilis;* flame this loopful of material; cool the inoculating loop and streak another complete plate.	3.1. It is better to use two separate plates for this test because *B. subtilis* is a spreading organism. This characteristic would give apparent erroneous results if the two parts of this procedure were done on one agar plate.
4. Using the divided plate (see Step 2), streak one half of the plate with a loopful of *M. smegmatis;* flame the inoculating loop; obtain a second loopful of culture of *M. smegmatis;* flame this loopful of material. Cool the inoculating loop and streak the second half of this plate.	4.1. *M. smegmatis* is not a spreader and the two halves of this plate should show different results.
5. Incubate all plates.	5.1. Consult your instructor about the place to be used for incubation.

KEY STEPS | **IMPORTANT POINTS**

B. *Dry Heat-Hot Air Oven:*

1. Obtain the Petri dishes which contain
    a. ½ cm gauze squares moistened with **B. subtilis**
    b. ½ cm gauze squares moistened with **S. aureus**
With sterile forceps, transfer one square from each of these Petri dishes to two different tubes of nutrient broth.

1.1. You will get better results if you transfer the square which has **S. aureus** on it first. Dip the tips of your forceps into a beaker with alcohol (about 5 cm high in the beaker), flame the tips of your forceps, let the alcohol burn in the air (this sterilizes the forceps), then transfer the gauze square which has been moistened with a culture of **S. aureus,** and again the one with **B. subtilis.** Label the tubes.
1.2. These tubes are your controls. Store them in the refrigerator and incubate them together with the nutrient agar tubes in Step 5.

2. Transfer a second ½ cm square of each of these cultures to the inside of two gauze squares (5 cm square).

2.1. The ½ cm gauze containing the culture of **S. aureus** should be placed in one 5 cm gauze square in the Petri dish and the gauze containing the culture of **B. subtilis** should be placed in a second 5 cm gauze square. Why?
2.2. Always make all transfers with a flame sterilized forceps (see Step 1.1.).

3. Wrap each 5 cm gauze square prepared in Step 2 in a separate wrapping. Label. See Steps 3.1., 3.2. (on the right), for this procedure.

3.1. The wrappings which may be used are double thickness muslin, special *dressing* wrapping or double thickness of *heavy brown paper.*
3.2. Why do you need to wrap these individually?
3.3. Why do they need to be labeled?

4. Place all wrapped materials (and organisms) in the *"cold"* hot air oven.

4.1. Let the instructor sterilize all materials in the hot air oven; they will be returned to you during the next laboratory period.
4.2. Sterilization occurs in the hot air oven for over 2 hr at 170-180 C. How long does it take for your oven to reach 170 C? How long does the oven take to cool off?
4.3. When can the sterile materials be removed from the oven?

5. After sterilization, unwrap carefully with sterile procedures; then using an alcohol flamed forceps, transfer each of the ½ cm gauze squares to two different tubes of nutrient broth. Label and incubate all tubes. Don't forget the controls from Step 1.

5.1. Why do you use a well flamed sterile forceps to transfer the gauze to the tubes of broth?
5.2. Should you have a separate sterile forceps for each of these organisms? When would this be necessary?

Record of Results:

1. Record all results on the chart provided.

EFFECT OF DRY HEAT ON BACTERIA*

Treatment	*B. subtilis*	*M. smegmatis*	*S. aureus*
Incineration			
Hot air oven			
Untreated control			

*Incubated after treatment as convenient.

Questions:

1. Another example of incineration than that used in this experiment is __________

__________.

2. The hot air oven can be used to sterilize __________,

__________, __________ and __________.

3. The temperature of boiling water (at sea level) is __________.

4. **Bacillus subtilis** was used in this experiment and Exercise 21 because __________

____

5. **Mycobacterium smegmatis** was used in this experiment and Exercise 21 because

__________.

6. **Staphylococcus aureus** was used in this experiment and Exercise 21 because__________

__________.

Laboratory Exercise 21

TOPIC: EFFECTS OF MOIST HEAT ON MICROORGANISMS

OBJECTIVES:
1. To show the effect of moist heat and pressurized steam on bacteria.
2. To show the relation of heat, as a physical agent of destruction of bacteria, to sterile technique.

EQUIPMENT:
1. Three 5 day broth cultures of *Bacillus subtilis.*
2. Three 5 day broth cultures of *Mycobacterium smegmatis.*
3. Three 48 hr broth cultures of *Staphylococcus aureus* (nonpathogenic strain).
4. Eight sterile nutrient agar Petri plates.
5. Eighteen sterile nutrient broth tubes.
6. 1½ cm gauze squares contaminated with a culture of *B. subtilis.*
7. 1½ cm gauze squares contaminated with a culture of *M. smegmatis.*
8. 1½ cm gauze squares contaminated with a culture of *S. aureus* (nonpathogenic strain).
9. Forceps.
10. Bed linen or bed sheets.

Procedure:

KEY STEPS	IMPORTANT POINTS
A. *Moist Heat—Boiling:*	
1. Place the tubes with the broth cultures of *B. subtilis, M. smegmatis* and *S. aureus* in a beaker of boiling water.	1.1. Be sure that the level of the water in the beaker comes up to the level of the broth culture in the tubes. The entire culture must be surrounded with boiling water.
2. Leave in the boiling water for 1 min.	2.1. Has the entire culture been exposed to the temperature of boiling water for 1 minute? Explain. 2.2. Is the temperature of boiling water the same in all parts of the world? Explain.
3. At the end of 1 min, remove the cultures from the beaker of boiling water and transfer a loopful of each into three different tubes of nutrient broth.	3.1. From your knowledge of the nature of these organisms, discuss their susceptibility to the temperature of boiling water.
4. Repeat the procedure with the *same* cultures for 1 more min. These cultures were immersed in boiling water for a total of 2 min. Again, transfer a loopful of each organism to nutrient broth. Repeat the same procedure for a total exposure to heat for 3 min and then for 5 min.	4.1. What is the value of these different time factors? 4.2. What are the relationships between this experiment and some procedures encountered in the hospital?
5. Label and incubate all tubes.	

| **KEY STEPS** | **IMPORTANT POINTS** |

B. *Moist Heat—Autoclave:*

1. Prepare four sterile nutrient agar plates. Divide two into halves with wax pencil marks on the bottoms of the dishes.

1.1. See Exercise 7.
1.2. These nutrient agar plates are best prepared before the start of the laboratory.

2. Streak one Petri dish (not divided into halves) with a loopful of the culture of *B. subtilis.* Streak one half of one of the divided Petri dishes with a loopful of *S. aureus.* Streak one half of the second divided Petri dish with a loopful of *M. smegmatis.*

2.1. Why is it important to use three different organisms?
2.2. What important differences are there among these three organisms?
2.3. Why were these cultures chosen as representatives in this experiment?

3. Autoclave all three broth cultures at 121 C (15-18 lb pressure) for 15 min. Streak the remaining plate with the autoclaved culture of *B. subtilis.* Streak the remaining halves of the divided Petri dishes with the autoclaved broth cultures of *S. aureus* and *M. smegmatis.*

3.1. Is the temperature or the pressure more important in sterilizing with the autoclave?
3.2. Be sure to streak *S. aureus* on the plate which has *S. aureus* on it before autoclaving, and *M. smegmatis* on its specific plate.
3.3. Would lowering the temperature of the autoclave change the results?

4. Repeat Steps 1 to 3, using the autoclave at 121 C for 5 min instead of 15 min. If your autoclave is set for 18 lb pressure, autoclave for only 2 min.

4.1. Is the time factor important? Why?

5. Prepare three large tightly bound bundles of sheets. In the center of one bundle, place the 1½ cm gauze squares contaminated with *B. subtilis.* In the center of the second bundle, place the 1½ cm gauze square contaminated with *S. aureus.* In the third bundle, place the square contaminated with *M. smegmatis.* Wrap each bundle tightly and autoclave at 121 C for 15 min.

5.1. How is this experiment related to hospital procedures?

6. Remove from the autoclave and place the gauze squares in tubes of broth.

6.1. Each square should be put in a different tube of broth.
6.2. Use an alcohol flamed forceps and sterile techniques to transfer the gauze squares.

KEY STEPS	**IMPORTANT POINTS**
7. Repeat Steps 5 and 6, using small bundles (one sheet in each), loosely bound and wrapped.	7.1. What principles of sterilization are being demonstrated?
8. Label and incubate all tubes.	

Record of Results:

1. Record all results on the chart provided.

EFFECT OF MOIST HEAT ON BACTERIA

Treatment	*B. subtilis*	*M. smegmatis*	*S. aureus*
Boiling 1 min			
Boiling 2 min			
Boiling 3 min			
Boiling 5 min			
Autoclave (121 C for 15 min)			
Autoclave (121 C for 5 min)*			
Autoclave (tightly bound sheets)			
Autoclave (loosely bound sheets)			

*For an 18 lb pressure autoclave, sterilize for only 2 min.

Questions:

1. *Bacillus subtilis* was used in this experiment because ______________________

____.

2. *Mycobacterium smegmatis* was used in this experiment because ______________

____.

3. *Staphylococcus aureus* was used in this experiment because ______________

____.

4. An autoclave can be used to sterilize _______________________________

____________________, ____________________ and _____________________________.

5. The principle behind the use of heat for sterilization is _______________________

____.

6. Three important things to remember about the use of the autoclave for sterilizing

are:

a.

b.

c.

Laboratory Exercise 22

TOPIC: CHEMICAL DISINFECTION

OBJECTIVES:
1. To illustrate the action of chemical disinfectants and antiseptics on bacteria.
2. To help the student understand that there are differences in the effectiveness of chemicals used as disinfectants.
3. To give the student an understanding of the basis for chemical disinfection.

EQUIPMENT:*
1. 5 day broth culture of *Bacillus subtilis.*
2. 24 hr broth culture of *Escherichia coli.*
3. 24 hr broth culture of *Staphylococcus aureus* (nonpathogenic strain).
4. 5 ml or 10 ml sterile pipettes.
5. 1 ml sterile pipettes.
6. Lactose broth in Durham fermentation tubes.
7. Lactose broth with 0.05% sodium thioglycollate in Durham tubes (for mercurial disinfectants).
8. Nutrient broth in tubes.
9. Nutrient broth with 0.05% sodium thioglycollate in tubes (for mercurial disinfectants).
10. Lysol or saponated solution of cresol, 0.2% and 2%.
11. Phenol solutions, 1:80 and 1:100.
12. A household detergent solution, diluted as recommended on the package.
13. Ethyl alcohol, 20%, 40% and 70%.
14. Bichloride of mercury, 1:5,000.
15. Hexachlorophene in a commercial product, 0.3%. (Note that pHisoHex contains 3%, thus would be used in a 1:10 dilution)†, or you may use pHisoDerm.
16. Solutions of tincture of iodine, 0.1% and 0.5%.
17. Hydrogen peroxide, 3%.
18. Sterile test tubes.
19. Sterile human or animal blood serum or sterile whole milk.

Procedure: **Different disinfectants** are assigned to **different members** of the class.

Note: It may help the student to understand the procedures of this experiment better if attention is directed toward the chart of results prior to starting the experiment.

KEY STEPS	**IMPORTANT POINTS**
1. Using a 10 ml sterile pipette, transfer 5 ml of assigned disinfectant to a sterile test tube.	1.1. Why is it essential to use sterile technique? 1.2. *Caution:* Do not suck the disinfectant into your mouth when you are drawing the disinfectant into the pipette. 1.3. Ask your instructor to demonstrate a propipette to you, or another device that does not require pipetting by mouth. 1.4. Propipette holders are attached to sterile pipettes when used in this type of experiment.

---

*The quaternary ammonium compounds (like Zephiran, Phemerol, etc.) have been omitted from this exercise because a good inhibitor which is simple to use is unavailable.

†Hexachlorophene-containing products like pHisoHex may be bought only with a physician's prescription.

KEY STEPS	**IMPORTANT POINTS**
2. Using a 1 ml sterile pipette, transfer 0.5 ml of a broth culture of *E. coli* to the tube prepared in Step 1.	2.1. This procedure is adapted from the standard phenol coefficient test. *E. coli* has been substituted for *Salmonella typhi*. 2.2. When broth cultures are transferred by pipette, it is important that you should not get the culture into your mouth. Your instructor will tell you if you should be pipetting by mouth or using a propipette. Control the level of the culture in the pipette so that drops do not escape from the tip before you transfer to the test tube. 2.3. Whatever technique you use here, it is important that you learn both methods of using a pipette.
3. After intervals of 1, 5, 10 and 15 min, transfer a loopful of the culture-disinfectant mixture to separate tubes of lactose broth. Two lactose broth tubes are kept for controls; they receive the organism, but *no* disinfectants.	3.1. Be sure to rotate the tube containing the test organism and disinfectant just before each transfer. Why? 3.2. Use thioglycollate lactose broth in the tests using *E. coli* and mercurial disinfectants. Thioglycollate inhibits the action of mercurial disinfectants. The other disinfectants listed under equipment are inhibited by dilution. Why is it important to be concerned with the inhibition of the action of the disinfectant?
4. Repeat Steps 1 to 3, using *S. aureus* and nutrient broth instead of *E. coli* and lactose broth.	4.1. Why are the concentrations of disinfectants in the test lower than those commonly used?
5. Repeat Steps 1 to 3, using *B. subtilis* and nutrient broth instead of *E. coli* and lactose broth.	5.1. What are the characteristics of the three organisms used in this experiment which are important from the viewpoint of disinfection?
6. Repeat steps 1 to 5, adding 1 ml of serum or sterile milk to the disinfectant before adding the broth culture. Do the same with three of the controls (the three different organisms).	6.1. Almost all disinfectants lose some of their effectiveness in the presence of protein. Why?
7. Incubate all tubes at 37 C for 24 hr.	

Record of Observations: The data are recorded by the students who used specific disinfectants. All class data are pooled.

1. Record the results on the chart provided. Show growth as +, indicating that the disinfectant did *not* kill the organism; no growth as 0, indicating that the disinfectant did kill the organism.

THE EFFECT OF DISINFECTANTS ON CULTURES OF BACTERIA

Disinfectants	E. coli				S. aureus				B. subtilis			
	min				min				min			
	1	5	10	15	1	5	10	15	1	5	10	15
Lysol, 0.2%												
Lysol, 0.2% with serum or milk												
Lysol, 2%												
Lysol, 2 % with serum or milk												
Phenol, 1:80												
Phenol, 1:80 with serum or milk												
Phenol, 1:100												
Phenol, 1:100 with serum or milk												
A household detergent*												
A household detergent with serum or milk												
Ethyl alcohol, 20%												
Ethyl alcohol, 20% with serum or milk												
Ethyl alcohol, 40%												
Ethyl alcohol, 40% with serum or milk												
Ethyl alcohol, 70%												
Ethyl alcohol, 70% with serum or milk												
Bichloride of mercury, 1:5,000												
Bichloride of mercury, 1:5,000 with serum or milk												
Hexachlorophene,† 0.3% (in pHisoHex)												
Hexachlorophene,† 0.3% (in pHisoHex) with serum or milk												
Solution of tincture of iodine, 0.1%												
Solution of tincture of iodine, 0.1% with serum or milk												
Solution of tincture of iodine, 0.5%												
Solution of tincture of iodine, 0.5% with serum or milk												
Hydrogen peroxide, 3%												
Hydrogen peroxide, 3% with serum or milk												
Control (without disinfectant)												
Control with serum or milk (no disinfectant)												

*Use the household detergent in the proportion recommended on the package (see Equipment 12.)
†Or pHisoDerm.

EFFECTS OF COMMONLY USED DISINFECTANTS*

Disinfectants	% Conc.	Activity on			
		Bacteria		Fungi	Viruses
		Vegetative cells	Spores		
Ethyl Alcohol	70–90	Good	None	Fair	Fair
Isopropyl alcohol	70–90	Very good	None	Good	Fair
Isopropyl alcohol—iodine	70 0.5–2.0	Very good	Fair	Good	Good
Formaldehyde solution, USP	37	Good	Good	Good	Good
Formaldehyde—alcohol	20 50	Very good	Very good	Good	Good
Phenolic compounds, cresols	1.0–5.0	Good	Poor	Good	Poor
Chlorine (hypochlorites)	1.0–5.0	Very good	Fair	Fair	Good
Glutaraldehyde	2.0	Very good	Very good	Good	Good
Iodine (aqueous)	2.0–5.0	Very good	Poor	Good	Good
Iodophors	1.00	Good	Poor	Poor	Good
Hexachlorophene	3.0–4.0	Fair	None	Good	Not known
Benzalkonium chloride (1:750–1:1,000)		Very good	None	Good	None
Ethylene oxide gas	Mixture	Very good	Good	Good	Good

*Adapted from The Medical Letter on Drugs and Therapeutics, copyright 1967.

Questions:

1. Hydrogen peroxide is a disinfectant because of its rapid release of _____________

   ____ in the presence of organic material.

2. Bichloride of mercury acts by ____ .

3. Tincture of iodine is effective as a disinfectant because it _________________

   ____ .

4. Ten important factors involved in chemical disinfection are:

   a.   f.

   b.   g.

   c.   h.

   d.   i.

   e.   j.

5. The tests of chemicals to be used in disinfection should be carried into practical
situations. Name three types of tests which could be done.

   a.

   b.

   c.

6. What is the difference between "naked" organisms and protected organisms?
   In disinfection procedures in the hospital are we usually concerned with "naked"
   or protected organisms?
   How does this affect procedures used?

7. What problems resulted from the use of hexachlorophene as a disinfectant in
   hospitals?

Laboratory Exercise 23

TOPIC: ACTION OF DYES AND ANTIBIOTICS

OBJECTIVES: 1. To show the inhibiting action of certain dyes and antibiotics on bacteria.
2. To give the student an understanding of the bacteriological basis of the use of these substances in the treatment of certain infectious diseases.

EQUIPMENT: 1. 24 hr broth culture of *Staphylococcus aureus* (nonpathogenic strain).
2. 24 hr broth culture of *Enterobacter aerogenes.*
3. 5 day broth culture of *Mycobacterium smegmatis.*
4. Crystal violet, 1:1,000, 1:10,000, 1:50,000 (same as gentian violet).
5. Sterile nutrient agar for plating.
6. Sterile Petri dishes.
7. Sterile 1 ml pipettes.
8. Forceps.
9. Disks containing various concentrations of antibiotics (Difco).

Procedure: The instructor may divide the antibiotics and dyes among members of the class; also, one individual may use only one organism. These results can then be compared and the class results pooled. Follow your instructor's directions.

KEY STEPS	IMPORTANT POINTS
1. To a tube of melted sterile nutrient agar which has been cooled to 45 C, add 1 ml of a 1:1,000 solution of crystal violet. Pour into a Petri dish and allow the agar to cool and harden.	1.1. When a solution is added to liquid agar medium, it is important not to cool the agar below 45 C before adding the solution. Why?
2. Prepare a second pour plate by adding 1 ml of a 1:10,000 solution of crystal violet to the melted and cooled nutrient agar.	2.1. How will bacteriostasis be evident with these three dilutions of dyes?
3. Prepare a third pour plate which contains 1 ml of a 1:50,000 solution of crystal violet.	
4. Mark the bottom of each Petri dish into four segments.	
5. Streak one segment on each plate with one of the test organisms. Repeat, using a second segment for the second test organism. Use the third segment for the third test organism and save one segment on each plate for the control.	5.1. What is the value of using these three test organisms in this experiment? 5.2. Be careful to stay within the lines when streaking the segments on the plates.
6. Label each plate and each segment carefully and incubate.	

KEY STEPS	**IMPORTANT POINTS**

7. To a tube of melted sterile nutrient agar which has been cooled to 45 C, add a loopful of a broth culture of **S. aureus.** Mix well, pour into a sterile Petri dish. Rotate the dish gently and allow the agar to cool and harden.

7.1. Why is it important to cool the nutrient agar to 45 C before adding the culture?

8. With alcohol flamed sterile forceps place disks of various concentrations of antibiotics on the agar surface of the plate.*

8.1. Six disks can be placed on each plate. This allows adequate space between the disks to observe zones of inhibition (see diagram).

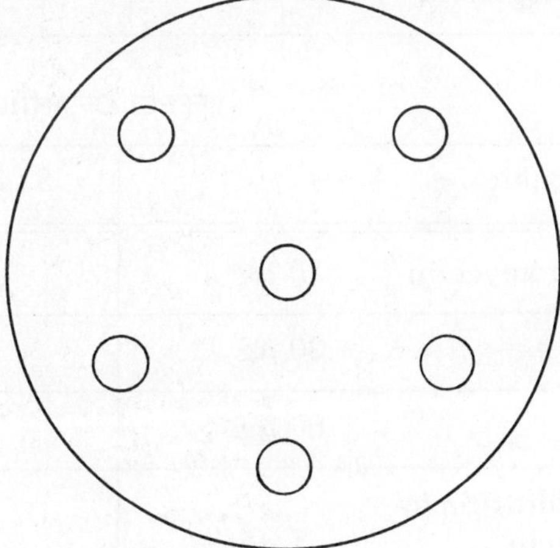

9. Make a second pour plate with **E. aerogenes** and place disks of the same concentrations of the same antibiotics used in Step 8.

10. Repeat Steps 7 and 8, using **M. smegmatis** as the test organism.

10.1. What are the advantages of using these three organisms in this experiment?

11. Label all plates and incubate them as directed.

11.1. Consult your instructor about a place for incubation. These plates should *not* be inverted. Why?

Difco manual, 9th ed. Difco Laboratories, Detroit, 1953, p. 337.

Record of Observations:

1. Record the amount and kind of growth of the organisms which have been in contact with crystal violet.
2. Measure from the outer edge of the clear zone across the disk to the outer edge of the clear zone on the other side. Record in millimeters the effects of all antibiotics.

EFFECT OF DYES ON BACTERIA

Organism Tested	Crystal Violet		
	1:1000	1:10,000	1:50,000
S. aureus			
E. aerogenes			
M. smegmatis			

EFFECT OF ANTIBIOTICS ON BACTERIA

Antibiotic*		*S. aureus*	*E. aerogenes*	*M. smegmatis*
Chloromycetin	10 μg			
	30 μg			
	60 μg			
Dihydrostrepto-mycin	1 μg			
	10 μg			
	100 μg			
Penicillin	0.5 unit			
	1 unit			
	10 units			
Polymyxin B	5 μg			
	10 μg			
	30 μg			
Terramycin	10 μg			
	30 μg			
	60 μg			

*Other antibiotics may be added or substituted at the discretion of the instructor.

EFFECT OF ANTIBIOTICS ON BACTERIA (CONTINUED)

Antibiotic		*S. aureus*	*E. aerogenes*	*M. smegmatis*
Aureomycin	10 μg			
	30 μg			
	60 μg			
Bacitracin	2 units			
	10 units			
	20 units			

Questions:

1. What is meant by bacteriostatic action? How does this apply to sulfonamides?

2. Fill in the following chart.

EFFECT OF ANTIBIOTICS ON SOME ORGANISMS CAUSING DISEASES

Antibiotic	Source	Organisms It Affects	Diseases in Which Used
Aureomycin			
Bacitracin			
Chloromycetin			
Dihydrostreptomycin			
Penicillin			
Polymyxin B			
Terramycin			
Achromycin			

3. Name five dyes other than crystal violet that could have been used in this experiment.

4. Name 10 antibiotics other than those used in this experiment.

Laboratory Exercise 24

TOPIC: DISINFECTION OF HANDS

OBJECTIVES:
1. To show the student commonly accepted methods for disinfection of hands to prevent transfer of disease.
2. To make the student conscious of the hands as a likely means of transfer of disease- and infection-causing microorganisms.

EQUIPMENT:*
1. 24 hr broth culture of *Serratia marcescens.*
2. Petri dish with gauze square contaminated with a few drops of broth culture of *S. marcescens.*
3. Sterile Petri dishes with strips of gauze in the bottom.†
4. Tubes of sterile nutrient agar (20 to 25 ml).
5. Tubes of sterile nutrient agar (20 to 25 ml) with 0.05% thioglycollate for cultures following disinfection with bichloride of mercury.
6. Aqueous Zephiran (benzalkonium chloride), 1:1,000, 1:2,000, 1:5,000.
7. Tincture Zephiran, 1:1,000, 1:2,000, 1:5,000.
8. Lysol, 1 per cent, 0.5%.
9. Bichloride of mercury, 1:1,000, 1:2,000, 1:5,000.
10. Ethyl alcohol, 70%.
11. pHisoHex or soap containing hexachlorophene, or pHisoDerm.
12. Sterile towels.
13. Sterile hand brushes.

Procedure: If all parts of this experiment are *not* done by all members of the class, it is most important that all students see how the experiments are done and observe the results.

KEY STEPS	IMPORTANT POINTS
For Preparing Cultures: 1. Melt tubes of sterile nutrient agar and cool to approximately 45 C. Pour a tube of agar into each Petri dish (which contains gauze strips) that is needed for your experiment. Allow the nutrient agar to harden.	1.1. Consult with instructor about the part or parts of this experiment that you should do.

---

*Other disinfectants than those listed may be added or substituted by the instructor.

†These are prepared by cutting gauze strips 2 cm wide. One set of these strips should be just long enough to lie flat on the bottom of the Petri dish. A second set of gauze strips should be long enough to extend up the sides of the Petri dish to make tabs. The strips of gauze are moistened and placed in the bottom of the Petri dish with the short strip on top of the longer one and at right angles to each other. The covers are placed on the Petri dishes and the dishes stacked on their sides in a large rectangular enamel pan. The Petri dishes are sterilized in the autoclave and used as soon as possible after sterilization.

KEY STEPS	**IMPORTANT POINTS**

2. While you hold the bottom of the Petri dish inverted over the fingers of your right hand, ask your partner to pull on the gauze tab on the side of the dish with a sterile forceps until the entire agar circle falls on your fingers. Return the circle of agar immediately to the bottom of the Petri dish and roll the tips of the fingers on end so that the tips of the fingers contact the agar.

2.1. If you are left handed, do the culture of your left hand.
2.2. This plate will show the normal inhabitants of your hand. (Control test No. 1.)
2.3. Be careful not to crack or break the agar.
2.4. On the bottom of the Petri dish indicate what area of agar was contaminated by your fingertips.

3. Contaminate the fingers of your right hand by handling the gauze square moistened with a few drops of broth culture of *S. marcescens.* Dry the fingers in the air.

3.1. This simulates handling contaminated materials.
3.2. *S. marcescens* is a good test organism for this experiment because _____________

____ ,

____ .

3.3. Why should you dry the fingers after contaminating them?

4. Make another culture from your fingers by following the directions in Step 2.

4.1. This culture will be the contaminated control.

5. Use the procedure for handwashing or disinfection assigned to you by your instructor. Follow the specific instructions given below.

For Hand Washing:
1. Contaminate the fingers of both hands with the gauze sponge moistened with a broth culture of *S. marcescens.* Dry the fingers in the air.

1.1. Why should you contaminate the fingers of both hands after streaking the plate for the contaminated control?

2. Wash your hands with soap and running water for an assigned time (½ min, 1 min, 1½ min, 2 min). Dry your hands with a sterile towel. Prepare a culture by following directions given in Step 2 under "For Preparing Cultures." Inoculate a plate for each hand. Label all plates and incubate them at room temperature.

2.1. Paper towels may have spores on them which would be transferred to your hands. These spores might germinate and produce growth on your plates and give confusing results.
2.2. *S. marcescens* will not produce its pigment at temperatures higher than 30 C.
2.3. Do not incubate these plates in an inverted position because the agar has been loosened from the bottom of the Petri dish and will fall to the cover if incubated upside down.

KEY STEPS	IMPORTANT POINTS

For Hand Scrubbing:

1. Follow the direction given in Step 1 under "For Hand Washing"

2. Scrub your hands with a sterile hand brush for an assigned time (1 min, 3 min, 5 min, 7 min). Dry your hands with a sterile towel and prepare cultures by following directions given in Step 2 under "For Preparing Cultures."

    2.1. What are the advantages of using a hand brush for scrubbing?
    2.2. What are the disadvantages of using a hand brush?

3. Repeat Steps 1 and 2 above under "For Hand Scrubbing." Instead of using a time factor, scrub each area for an assigned number of times (once, three times, five times).

    3.1. When scrubbing hands, is it more important to watch the clock or to observe the areas that you have scrubbed? Why?

4. Repeat directions for hand scrubbing, using pHisoHex or soap containing hexachlorophene, or use pHisoDerm.

    4.1. What is hexachlorophene?
    4.2. What are the advantages of using a soap containing hexachlorophene? Disadvantages?
    4.3. What is pHisoDerm?

For Soaking Hands in a Disinfectant:

1. Obtain a basin or suitable container for the disinfectant assigned to you. Pour in enough disinfectant to cover your hand when you are ready to use it. After preparing plates as directed under "For Preparing Cultures," recontaminate the fingers of your right hand (left hand for left handed students). Dry the fingers in the air.

    1.1. What are the advantages of using a disinfectant for contaminated hands?
    1.2. What are the disadvantages of using a disinfectant for contaminated hands?

2. Place the contaminated fingers in the disinfectant for the assigned time (½ min, 1 min, 1½ min, 2 min). Gently rinse off the disinfectant with tap water. Dry the hand with a sterile towel. Label all plates and incubate them at 20 to 25 C.

    2.1. Why is it important to rinse off the disinfectant in this experiment?

Record of Observations:

1. Record the results of your tests and the ones done by all other members of your laboratory section. Some colonies of **S. marcescens** may have lost almost all of their color after the organism was subjected to soap or disinfectants. Look at all colonies very carefully to observe the slight pink color or the pink centers on some of these colonies.

CONTROL RESULTS FOR HAND WASHING, HAND SCRUBBING AND DISINFECTION OF HANDS

Controls	Amount of Growth*	Presence of **S. marcescens**
Normal Inhabitants		
Contaminated Control		

The above table serves as control for the rest of the experiment (see pp. 119 and 120). All of the above squares should show growth.

*Indicate the amount of growth as +, 2+, 3+, 4+.

Instructions: In columns 1 indicate the amount of growth as +, 2+, 3+, 4+.
In columns 2 indicate by pos. or neg. whether or not any of the growth was **S. marcescens.**

RESULTS OF HAND WASHING WITH DISINFECTANTS USING DIFFERENT METHODS, TESTED ON *Serratia marcescens*

	½ min		1 min		1½ min		2 min		3 min		5 min		7 min	
	1	2	1	2	1	2	1	2	1	2	1	2	1	2
Hand Washing														
Hand Scrubbing (with Ordinary Soap)														
Hand Scrubbing (with Soap Containing Hexachlorophene, or pHisoHex or pHisoDerm)														
Hand Soaking: Aqueous Zephiran, 1:1,000														
Aqueous Zephiran, 1:2,000														
Aqueous Zephiran, 1:5,000														
Tincture Zephiran, 1:1,000														
Tincture Zephiran, 1:2,000														
Tincture Zephiran, 1:5,000														
Lysol, 1%														
Lysol, 0.5%														
HgCl$_2$, 1:1,000														
HgCl$_2$, 1:2,000														
HgCl$_2$, 1:5,000														
Ethyl alcohol, 70%														

TEST FOR EFFECTIVENESS OF HAND SCRUBBING

	One Stroke Count per Area		Three Stroke Counts per Area		Five Stroke Counts per Area	
	1	2	1	2	1	2
Hand Scrubbing (Stroke Count)						

Questions:

1. Define:

   a. Control

   b. Detergent

2. Give three reasons why **Serratia marcescens** is a desirable test organism for this experiment.

   a.

   b.

   c.

3. Why was the maximum time limited to 2 min for hand washing and disinfection of hands with chemicals?

4. Why was the scrubbing time increased to 7 min?

5. Why were these chemical substances chosen for an experiment on hand disinfection?

6. Discuss the importance of hand washing in the hospital.

Laboratory Exercises 25 to 27 have been designed for students who are using hospital facilities. They are not suited for college or university laboratories. Since these experiments are of a very practical nature, it is advised that all students should understand the purpose of these exercises whether or not they are being conducted in the students' own laboratories.

Laboratory Exercise 25

TOPIC: DISINFECTION OF THERMOMETERS

OBJECTIVES:
1. To show the student methods used in the disinfection of thermometers.
2. To make the student conscious of the importance of adequate disinfection of thermometers in the prevention of transfer of certain diseases.

EQUIPMENT:
1. Sterile glucose broth.
2. Sterile glucose broth with 0.05% sodium thioglycollate.
3. Sterile lactose broth in Durham fermentation tubes.
4. Sterile lactose broth with 0.05% sodium thioglycollate in Durham tubes.
5. Sterile, water-soluble lubricant for rectal thermometers.
6. Sterile petroleum jelly in covered containers.
7. Sterile glass rods 2 to 3 mm × 100 mm (approximately).
8. Sterile thermometer jars or small sterile enamel dishes.
9. Formalin, 4%.
10. Bichloride of mercury, 1:1,000 and 1:2,000.
11. Iodine, 0.5 per cent in 70% ethyl alcohol.
12. Iodine, 1.0 per cent in 70% ethyl alcohol.
13. Ethyl alcohol, 50 per cent, 70%, 95%.
14. Lysol, 1 per cent and 5%.
15. Tincture of green soap mixed with equal parts of 95% ethyl alcohol.
16. Sterile cotton balls.
17. Sterile water.
18. Specimen of thick mucus or sputum (not from patient who has tuberculosis).
19. Specimen of feces (not from patient who has an enteric infection).
20. Sterile Petri dishes.
21. Sterile forceps (or alcohol and flame to sterilize as needed).

Procedure:

KEY STEPS	IMPORTANT POINTS
For Oral Thermometers*: 1. Contaminate eight sterile glass rods with a thin film of mucus. Handle the contaminated glass rods with a sterile forceps	1.1. Why should you handle the contaminated glass rods with a forceps?
2. Transfer the contaminated glass rods to a sterile Petri dish and dry them by placing them in an incubator (37 C) for 30 min.	2.1. Drying the mucus on the glass rods simulates a hospital situation in which thermometers may not be disinfected immediately after temperatures are taken.

*Use sterile glass rods instead of thermometers so that you can sterilize them either in an autoclave or in a hot air oven.

KEY STEPS	IMPORTANT POINTS
3. Remove the Petri dish containing the glass rods from the incubator and transfer one contaminated rod to a tube of glucose broth.	3.1. Why should you use glucose broth for this test?
4. Place one contaminated glass rod in a container with the assigned disinfectant for 1 min.	4.1. It is important that the glass rod should be totally immersed in the disinfectant. Why?
5. Using a sterile forceps, remove a glass rod from the disinfectant and rinse it gently with sterile water.	5.1. Why is it important to use a sterile forceps here? 5.2. Why should you rinse the disinfected glass rod with water?
6. Place the disinfected and rinsed glass rod in a tube of glucose broth.	6.1. If your disinfectant is bichloride of mercury, use thioglycollate broth to inhibit the action of this disinfectant.
7*. Remove another glass rod from the Petri dish (see Step 2) and wash it with the tincture of green soap solution. Rinse it gently with sterile water and place this glass rod in a tube of glucose broth.	7.1. What are the reasons for washing thermometers with soap and water before disinfection?
8. Wash a third contaminated glass rod with soap and water, rinse, and place it in the assigned disinfectant for 1 min. Remove it from the disinfectant, rinse with sterile water and place the glass rod in a tube of glucose broth. Label all tubes and incubate at 37 C.	8.1. Why should these cultures be incubated at 37 C?
9. Repeat Steps 4, 5, 6, 8, increasing the disinfection time in Steps 4 and 8 to 2 min.	9.1. It is not necessary to repeat Step 7.
10. Repeat Steps 4, 5, 6, 8, increasing the disinfection time to 3 min.	10.1. What is the time for disinfection of thermometers that is recommended in most hospitals?
11. Repeat Steps 4, 5, 6, 8, increasing the disinfection time to 5 min.	

---

*If time is available, an additional series can be profitably included by substituting a dry cotton wipe for the soap wipe.

KEY STEPS	IMPORTANT POINTS

For Rectal Thermometers

1. Lubricate eight sterile glass rods with a thin film of a water-soluble lubricant. Contaminate these glass rods with a thin film of feces. Place one contaminated glass rod in a tube of lactose broth.

1.1. Water-soluble lubricants are sometimes called "surgical" lubricants.
1.2. If the water-soluble lubricant contains a mercurial disinfectant, use lactose broth which contains sodium thioglycollate.
1.3. The drying is omitted from this test because rectal thermometers are usually disinfected immediately after use.

2. Using a sterile forceps, wash one lubricated and contaminated glass rod with the tincture of green soap solution, rinse, and place in the disinfectant for 1 min. Remove from the disinfectant with a sterile forceps, rinse with sterile water and insert the glass rod in a tube of lactose broth. Label all tubes and incubate at 37 C.

2.1. Because it is customary to wash all rectal thermometers before disinfection, no tests are included here without this step.
2.2. If either the lubricant or the disinfectant contains a mercurial compound, use lactose broth with sodium thioglycollate.
2.3. Why should you use lactose broth for testing with these glass rods?

3. Repeat Step 2 with glass rods contaminated with feces, increasing the disinfection time to 2 min.

4. Repeat Step 2 in this series, increasing the disinfection time to 3 min.

5. Repeat Step 2 in this series increasing the disinfection time to 5 min.

6. Repeat Steps 1 to 5, using sterile petroleum jelly instead of the water-soluble lubricant.

6.1. What are the physical and chemical differences between water-soluble lubricant and petroleum jelly?
6.2. Would you expect to be able to remove petroleum jelly from a thermometer with soap and cold water? Why?

Results:

ORAL THERMOMETERS

INSTRUCTIONS: Under control, record the results of the test with the contaminated glass rod in glucose broth. Record whether there was growth or not after the various disinfection times. Record growth with a "+", no growth with "−".

	Control	No Wiping Before Disinfection				Soap Wiping Before Disinfection			
		1 min	2 min	3 min	5 min	1 min	2 min	3 min	5 min
Formalin, 4%									
Bichloride of mercury, 1:1,000									
Bichloride of mercury, 1:2,000									
Iodine, 0.5% in alcohol									
Iodine, 1.0% in alcohol									
Ethyl alcohol, 50%									
Ethyl alcohol, 70%									
Ethyl alcohol, 95%									
Lysol, 1%									
Lysol, 5%									

RECTAL THERMOMETERS

INSTRUCTIONS: Under control, record the results of the test with the contaminated glass rod in lactose broth. Under the time, record growth with a "+", no growth with "−", acid and gas with "⊕".

	Control	Water-soluble Lubricant				Petroleum Jelly as a Lubricant			
		1 min	2 min	3 min	5 min	1 min	2 min	3 min	5 min
Formalin, 4%									
Bichloride of mercury, 1:1,000									
Bichloride of mercury, 1:2,000									
Iodine, 0.5% in alcohol									
Iodine, 1.0% in alcohol									
Ethyl alcohol, 50%									
Ethyl alcohol, 70%									
Ethyl alcohol, 95%									
Lysol, 1%									
Lysol, 5%									

Questions:

1. Would dried mucus be harder or easier to remove from thermometers than moist mucus?

    Why?

2. What diseases might be transferred by means of the mouth thermometer?

3. What diseases might be transferred by means of the rectal thermometer?

4. Is it desirable to allow such a short time as 5 min for disinfection of thermometers with some disinfectants?

Which disinfectants?

5. What organisms might be present in sputum which were not included in this exercise?

Would you expect them to be more or less resistant than those used in this experiment?

Why?

6. What organisms might be present in feces which were not included in this exercise?

Would you expect them to be more or less resistant than those used in this experiment?

Why?

Laboratory Exercise 26

TOPIC: PREVENTION OF TRANSFER OF ORGANISMS CAUSING INFECTIONS FROM CONTAMINATED DRESSINGS

OBJECTIVES: 1. To show the student why and how to prevent contamination of hands when handling contaminated dressings.

EQUIPMENT: 1. Surgical dressing from an infected wound (from a patient who is not on antibiotic therapy).*
2. Sterile nutrient agar in tubes for plating.
3. Sterile Petri dishes.
4. Sterile Petri dishes with gauze strips (see Exercise 24).
5. Sterile brain heart infusion broth in tubes.
6. Sterile forceps.
7. Sterile towels.

Procedure:

KEY STEPS	IMPORTANT POINTS
For Handling Dressing with Hands: †	
1. Prepare three sterile nutrient agar plates according to instructions given in Exercise 24.	
2. Invert one nutrient agar plate over the fingers of the right hand. Use the gauze tab to pull the circle of agar onto the fingers. Return the circle of agar to the bottom of the Petri dish.	2.1. This is the control for normal inhabitants. 2.2. Your partner can help you by pulling the circle of agar down on your fingers.
3. Contaminate the fingers of one hand by handling the dressing from the infected wound. Inoculate the second agar plate with the fingers of the contaminated hand.	3.1. This is the contaminated control. 3.2. Use the inoculating procedure described in Exercise 24.
4. Wash both hands carefully with soap and running water, using extra friction on the contaminated fingers. Dry the hands with a sterile towel. Inoculate the third agar plate with the fingers of the hand contaminated in Step 3.	

---

*If this cannot be obtained, moisten gauze well with one of the following cultures: **Staphylococcus**

†CAUTION: This experiment ***should not be done*** by anyone who has cuts, abrasions or hangnails on any fingers of the right hand (for a right handed person), or on the left hand for a left-handed person.

KEY STEPS	**IMPORTANT POINTS**
5. Label all plates and incubate with the cover of the Petri dish on top.	5.1. See Exercise 24.
6. Prepare gram-stained smears of different colonies from both Petri dishes.	6.1. Examine smears with the microscope.

For Handling Dressings with Forceps:

KEY STEPS	**IMPORTANT POINTS**
1. Pick up contaminated dressing with sterile forceps. Return the dressing to its container.	1.1. If sterile forceps are not available, dip the tips of the forceps in alcohol and flame the tips in the flame of a Bunsen burner.
2. Immerse the tips of the forceps in a tube of broth. Label and incubate this culture.	2.1. Flame the tips of the forceps again, as in 1.1., or return the forceps to its container and sterilize by autoclaving.
3. After incubation, prepare a gram-stained smear from this culture.	3.1. See Exercise 9. 3.2. Examine the smear with the microscope.

Record of Observations:

1. Record results of these tests in the spaces provided.

RESULTS OF HANDLING CONTAMINATED DRESSINGS

Cultures of Hands	Number of Colonies	Description of Colonies	Morphology and Gram Stain
Normal inhabitants			
Contaminated hands			
Hands after washing			

Culture of Forceps:

Amount of growth

Result of the Gram stain

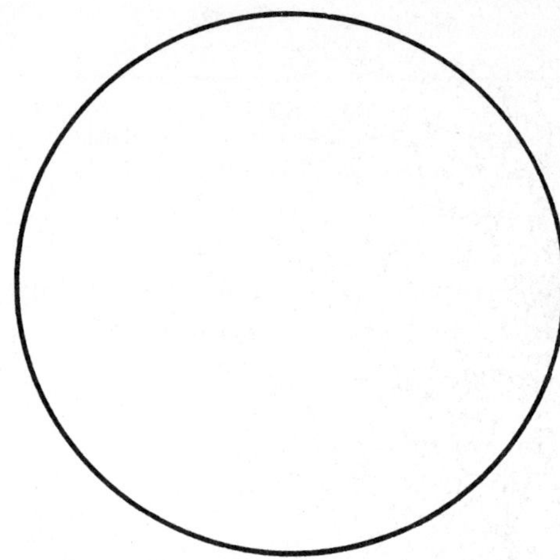

Questions:

1. Four organisms other than **Staphylococcus aureus** which can become contaminants of wounds are:

   a.

   b.

   c.

   d.

2. Why should you always avoid handling contaminated dressings with your hands? Discuss fully.

3. Why should you always avoid handling contaminated dressings with a transfer forceps that is going to be used to procure sterile dressings or instruments from general supply? Discuss fully.

4. How would you sterilize forceps which have handled contaminated dressings from a wound infected with **S. aureus?** With **Clostridium perfringens?** Why should these be handled differently?

Laboratory Exercise 27

TOPIC: CLEANING AND STERILIZING RUBBER CATHETERS AND RECTAL TUBES

OBJECTIVES: 1. To show the student methods of sterilizing catheters and other tubes.
2. To demonstrate safe methods of sterilizing rubber or plastic tubing without unnecessary damage and deterioration of the tubing.

EQUIPMENT: 1. Sterile rubber or plastic catheters and rectal tubes.
2. Voided specimen of urine (24 hr old).
3. 24 hr broth culture of *Escherichia coli* (add to the urine specimen).
4. Specimen of feces diluted with small amount of water in a wide-mouthed bottle to make a semiliquid suspension.
5. Sterile lactose broth in Durham tubes.
6. Sterilizer or container in which tubes can be boiled.
7. Container in which tubes can be soaked in a disinfectant.
8. Lysol, 1 per cent (other disinfectants may be used if desired).
9. Sterile towels.
10. Sterile transfer forceps.

Procedure:

KEY STEPS	IMPORTANT POINTS
For Catheters: 1. Contaminate the tip of a sterile rubber or plastic catheter by dipping it 2 or 3 inches into the specimen of urine. Inoculate a tube of lactose broth with the contaminated tip of the catheter.	1.1. Why was a culture of *E. coli* added to the specimen of urine?
2. Wash the catheter thoroughly with soap and running water. Rinse thoroughly. Inoculate a second tube of lactose broth with the tip of the contaminated catheter.	
3. Boil the catheter in a sterilizer or container for 1 min. Remove the catheter from the boiling water, drain the catheter completely and place it on a sterile towel until it is cool enough to handle.	3.1. Be sure that the entire catheter is immersed in the boiling water. Why? 3.2. Why should you drain any tubing thoroughly before placing it on a sterile surface?
4. When the catheter is cool enough to handle, inoculate a third tube of lactose broth with the tip of the catheter. Label and incubate all tubes.	
5. Repeat Steps 1 to 4, increasing the boiling time to 2 min.	

KEY STEPS	IMPORTANT POINTS
6. Repeat Steps 1 to 4, increasing the boiling time to 3 min.	
7. Repeat Steps 1 to 4, increasing the boiling time to 5 min.	7.1. What happens to rubber or plastic tubing that has been boiled too long? 7.2. There are different types of plastic tubing. You should know what type you are using.
8. Repeat Steps 1 to 7, omitting the washing of the catheter with soap and water.	
9. Repeat Steps 1 and 2 and autoclave the catheter at 121 C for 5 min.	9.1. What precautions must be taken if you autoclave rubber or plastic tubing? 9.2. Note that there are different types of plastics. Some may be autoclaved, while others may not. Why?
10. Repeat Step 9, omitting the washing of the catheter with soap and water.	
11. Repeat Steps 1 to 8, but substitute a disinfectant for the boiling water.	11.1. What effects do some disinfectants have on tubing?

For Rectal Tubes:

1. Contaminate the tip of a rectal tube by dipping it 2 to 3 inches into the specimen of feces. Inoculate a tube of lactose broth with the contaminated tip of the rectal tube.

2. Follow the instructions just given for catheters.

Record of Observations:

1. Record all results on the table provided. Look for cloudiness of the broth and gas production. Indicate no growth as "−", growth as "+" and gas produced as "⊕".

RESULTS OF CLEANING AND STERILIZING CATHETERS AND RECTAL TUBES

Tests		Catheters Lactose Broth		Rectal Tubes Lactose Broth	
		Growth	Gas	Growth	Gas
Contaminated Control					
Washing					
After Washing: Boil	1 min				
	2 min				
	3 min				
	5 min				
Autoclave	5 min				
Disinfectant	1 min				
	2 min				
	3 min				
	5 min				
No Washing: Boil	1 min				
	2 min				
	3 min				
	5 min				
Autoclave	5 min				
Disinfectant	1 min				
	2 min				
	3 min				
	5 min				

Questions:

1. Is it usually essential to have sterile rectal tubes for nursing procedures requiring this equipment? Why?

2. Is it essential to have sterile rubber catheters for catheterization? Why?

3. This procedure has checked primarily for one group of microorganisms. Why?

4. What pathogenic microorganisms might be found in urine?

5. What pathogenic microorganisms might be found in feces?

Unit 3

EXPERIMENTS SHOWING SOME SOURCES OF INFECTION, AND DEMONSTRATIONS OF IMMUNIZING AGENTS

The hospital personnel must always recognize that they have a distinct obligation to protect patients from infections. Hands, instruments, utensils and all other objects must be scrupulously clean and, in some instances, instruments and utensils must be sterile before coming into contact with patients. In general, the resistance of sick people is lower than that of healthy people to both general and specific infections. A review of the experiments included in Unit II should emphasize the importance of hand washing, thermometer disinfection, adequate decontamination of instruments, proper cleaning and disinfection of catheters and rectal tubes, and should also point out other implications in preventing infection by nursing procedures which are carried out with thorough understanding and application of microbiological principles.

Nurses, physicians, medical technologists, attendants and other health personnel not only have a responsibility for doing what are commonly considered their procedures, but also must frequently assume responsibility for, or at least have an understanding of, other objects or substances which may transfer infectious organisms. Food, water and insects may play a role in the transfer of pathogenic organisms from person to person. These factors are considered in this unit. Fomites as transmitting agents, and dirt in any form, must never be overlooked, especially in the hospital situation.

TOPIC: PREVENTION OF INFECTION WITH VACCINES, TOXOIDS, ANTISERA AND ANTITOXINS

The hospital personnel have a distinct responsibility to the public to promote immunization against specific infections. Therefore, health workers need to have a thorough understanding of the immunizing agents available, how they are administered, when they should be given, and what results can be expected from their use.

Briefly, immunizing agents can be divided into two groups, i.e., those which contain antibodies and provide some protection against a specific organism for short periods of time, or those that (as in vaccinations) produce an actual subclinical infection due to an active agent of disease, or its products. The latter type of immunization may be of longer duration. Physicians and nurses play an important role in educating the public, assisting with and, in some instances, carrying out immunization programs and frequently determining when immunization is imperative. People in contact with patients should also remember to take advantage of these immunizing agents in maintaining and promoting their own personal health programs.

Laboratory Exercise 28

TOPIC: BACTERIAL POLLUTION OF SEWAGE

OBJECTIVES: 1. To show bacterial pollution of sewage.
2. To demonstrate methods of isolating and differentiating certain members of the intestinal bacteria (Enterobacteriaceae).
3. To impress the student with the importance of good sewage disposal in preventing the transfer of infectious diseases of the intestinal tract.

EQUIPMENT: 1. Specimen of feces mixed in prescription bottle with water to give a thin suspension.*
2. Sterile tubes of lactose broth in Durham fermentation tubes.
3. Sterile 1 ml pipettes.
4. Sterile Eosin Methylene Blue Agar (EMB agar) in tubes for plating.
5. Sterile Petri dishes.
(Note: EMB agar plates may be prepared in advance, instead of using equipment 4 and 5).
6. Bacto XLD Agar plates (Xylose Lysine Agar with sodium desoxycholate, sodium thiosulfate and ferric ammonium citrate).

Procedure:

KEY STEPS	**IMPORTANT POINTS**
1. With a sterile 1 ml pipette transfer 0.1 ml of the dilution of sewage to a tube of lactose broth. Label the tube and incubate at 37 C.	1.1. Be careful in pipetting so that you do not get this material in your mouth. Again, your instructor will advise you if you should be pipetting by mouth or using a propipette.
2. After a minimum of 24 hr but not more than 48 hr of incubation, transfer a loopful of this culture to a plate of EMB agar. Spread the inoculum over the surface of the agar so that you will be likely to get isolated colonies.	2.1. EMB agar plates are prepared in the same way that other agar plates are prepared. 2.2. EMB agar contains eosin and methylene blue. These dyes are inhibitory to gram-positive organisms.
3. Transfer another loopful to an XLD Agar plate by the same procedure.	3.1. Bacto XLD Agar is designed for the direct isolation of **Shigella** and **Proteus inconstans**† from stool specimens. Look for red colonies. Some other **Proteus** strains will give black centered colonies on this medium. **Pseudomonas** may give a false positive red. **Escherichia, Klebsiella, Citrobacter, Enterobacter** and others produce yellow colonies.
4. Label each plate and incubate at 37 C for 24 to 48 hr.	4.1. Incubate the plates in the usual inverted position.
5. At the next laboratory period, inoculate tubes of lactose broth with material from two different isolated colonies from the EMB agar plate.	

---

  *Prescription bottles are easily available from pharmacies; they are inexpensive, autoclave well and make ideal dilution bottles. The 8 oz size is most convenient.
  †Previously referred to as the genus *Providencia*.

Record of Observations:

1. Record all results in the table provided.
2. Describe colonies found on EMB agar.
3. Describe the colonies found on XLD agar.

RESULTS OF TESTS ON SEWAGE

The lactose broth showed: no acid (no color change of indicator) ☐ − ; some acid ☐ ± ; acid (complete color change) ☐ + ; acid and gas ⊕ .

The EMB colonies were ☐ red ☐ purple ☐ with green metallic sheen ☐ all of these .

The XLD colonies were ☐ red ☐ yellow ☐ black centered ☐ other .

TESTS ON ISOLATED COLONIES

Isolated Colonies	Description	Fermentation in Lactose Broth
No. 1 from EMB		
No. 2 from EMB		
No. 3 from XLD		
No. 4 from XLD		

Questions:

1. What does the presence of coliform organisms in a sample of water indicate?

2. State two ways that cities use to dispose of their sewage adequately.

   a.

   b.

3. What precautions should be taken in disposing of feces from a patient who has typhoid fever?
   Why?

4. Why should a well be located on ground above the sewage disposal unit on a farm?

5. What are the dangers of emptying untreated sewage in any natural stream of water or harbor?

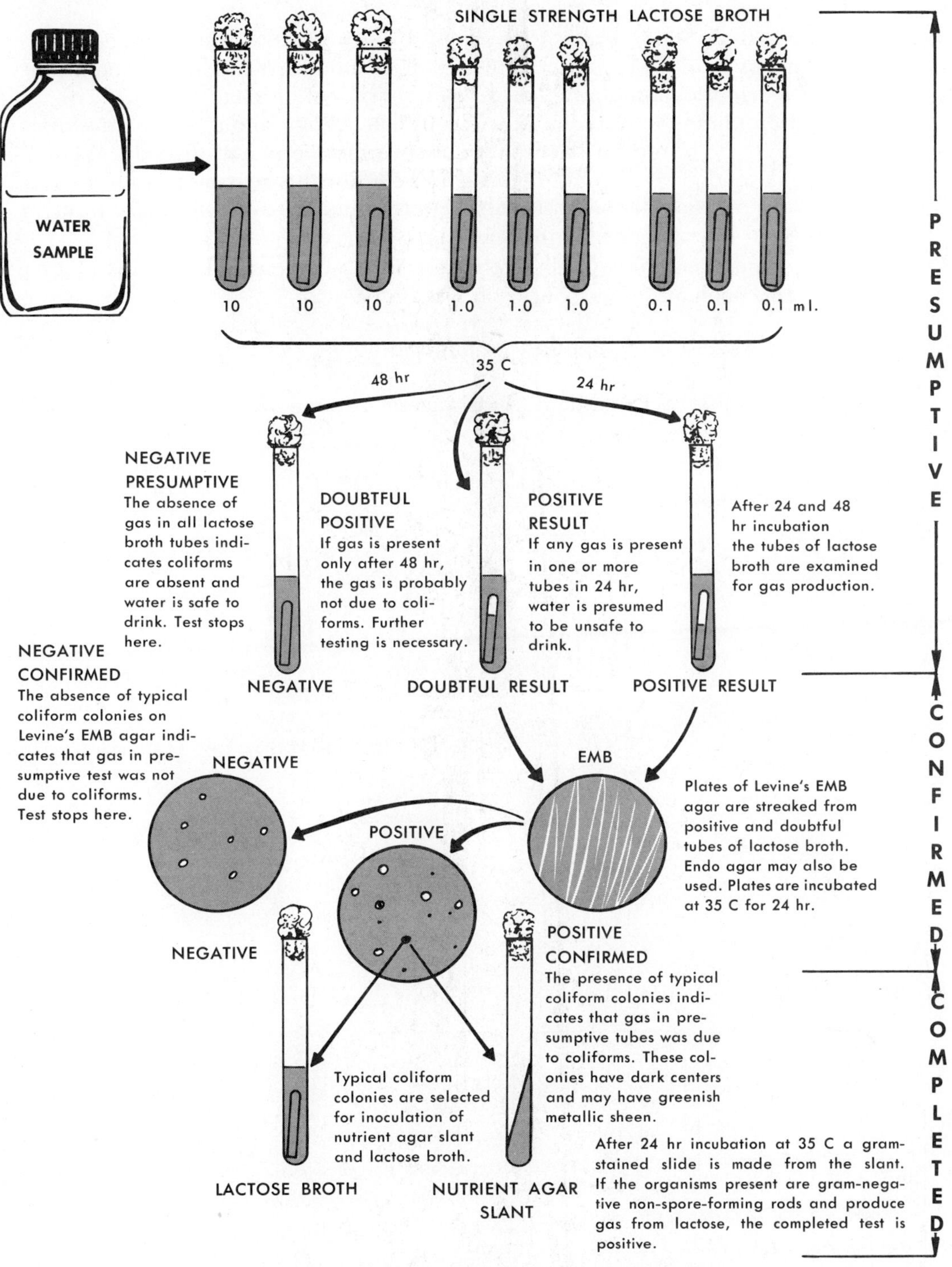

Bacteriological analysis of water as done routinely in many laboratories

TOPIC: METHODS AND PROCEDURES EMPLOYED IN WATER ANALYSIS

1. A method of routine water analysis has been perfected to test for coliform organisms in many laboratories which are water purification and community health oriented. Such a typical scheme is shown on page 129.
2. Dilution plating is important in water bacteriology but also any time the sample to be tested for bacterial counts cannot be plated directly. When a plate is seeded you cannot count colonies. For this reason dilution methods are very practical laboratory tools to determine the *most probable number* (MPN) of microorganisms in a sample. See next page.
3. The colonies on Petri plates are determined most easily by means of a colony counter. Such an instrument is shown on page 25.

Dilution Plating Methods

The dilution is first pipetted to the Petri plates. The medium (cool enough) is added later. See Exercise 29 for technique.

A. 10 ml dilution method:

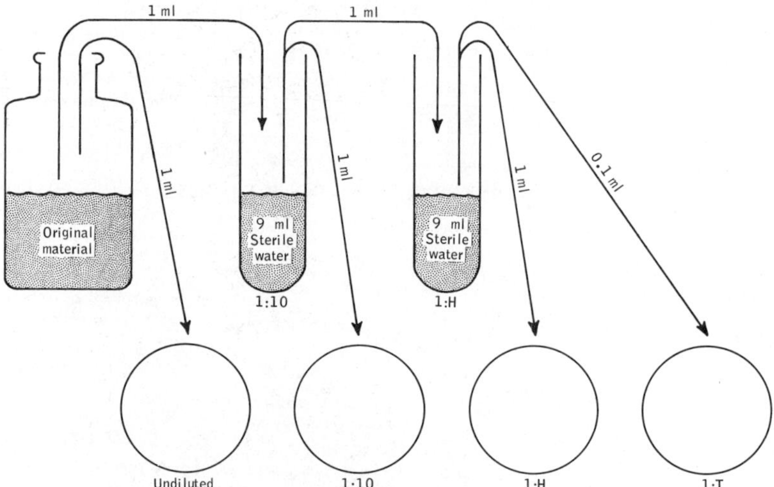

B. 100 ml bottle dilution method:

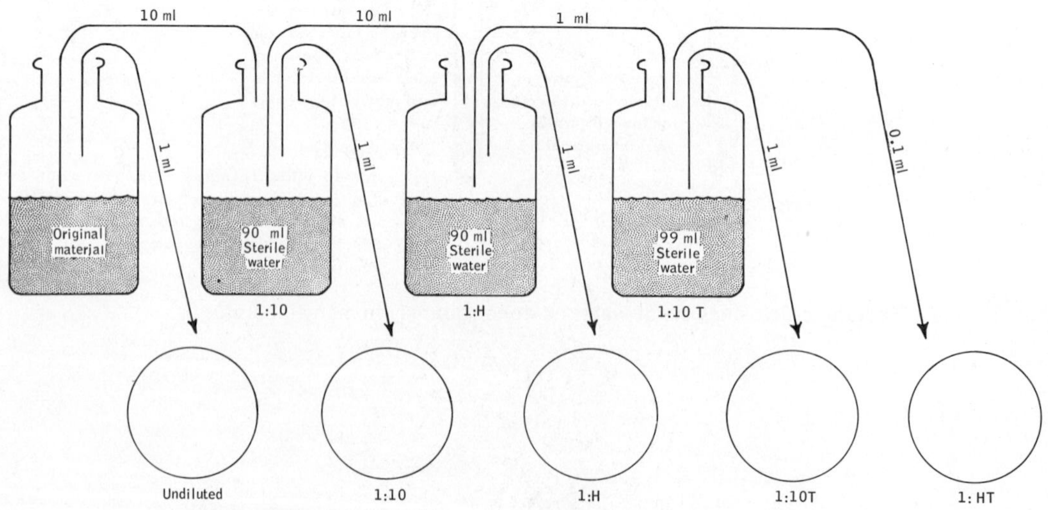

C. Statistical accuracy in counting of colonies:

The Committee on Standard Methods of the American Public Health Association recommends that the following table be used:

From   1 to   50 shall be recorded as found
From   51 to   100 shall be recorded to the nearest   5
From   101 to   250 shall be recorded to the nearest   10
From   251 to   500 shall be recorded to the nearest   25
From   501 to   1,000 shall be recorded to the nearest   50
From   1,001 to   10,000 shall be recorded to the nearest   100
From   10,001 to   50,000 shall be recorded to the nearest   500
From   50,001 to   100,000 shall be recorded to the nearest   1,000
From   100,001 to   500,000 shall be recorded to the nearest   10,000
From   500,001 to   1,000,000 shall be recorded to the nearest   50,000
From   1,000,001 to   10,000,000 shall be recorded to the nearest 100,000

For example if your plate count is 283, this is recorded as 275, or 82 becomes 80, and so forth. Counts below 30 and above 300 colonies per plate are not considered reliable.

Laboratory Exercise 29

TOPIC: BACTERIOLOGY OF WATER

OBJECTIVES:
1. To show some of the types of organisms found in water from different sources.
2. To demonstrate the importance of water purification and/or assurance of a safe source of water.

EQUIPMENT:
1. Samples of water from spring, well, river, swimming pool, city tap water supply.
2. Sterile 10 ml pipettes.
3. Sterile 1 ml pipettes, at least four for each water sample.
4. Sterile test tubes.
5. Sterile Petri dishes, at least four for each water sample.
6. Sterile nutrient agar for plating.
7. Sterile distilled water, at least four 9 ml water blanks for each water sample.
8. Sterile lactose broth (an indicator is not needed in this medium, for this purpose, since any gas indicates acid and gas production) in Durham tubes (at least five tubes for each water sample).
9. Sterile EMB agar plates for all water samples.
10. Gram's stain and slides.

Procedure: See the **dilution scheme drawings** and other methods on the pages following Exercise 28.

KEY STEPS	IMPORTANT POINTS
First Tests:	
1. With a sterile 1 ml pipette transfer 1 ml of sample to a sterile Petri dish. Transfer another 1 ml of the sample with the same pipette to a tube of lactose broth. Pour the melted nutrient agar (cooled to 45 C) into the Petri dish and rotate gently to mix the agar thoroughly with the water sample. Allow the agar to cool and harden. Label the plate and incubate the plate and tube of lactose broth at 37 C for 48 hr.	1.1. Be sure that the sample is mixed thoroughly just before transferring to the Petri dish and lactose broth. Why? 1.2. Why should you thoroughly mix the sample of water with the nutrient agar? 1.3. Why should these cultures be incubated at 37 C? 1.4. Under actual testing conditions five test tubes with lactose broth (Durham tubes) could be used in place of the one tube requested here for the undiluted sample. Each tube receives 1 ml water sample.
2. With a sterile 10 ml pipette, transfer 9 ml of sterile distilled water to a sterile, dry test tube. With a sterile 1 ml pipette, add 1 ml of the sample. Prepare cultures of this 1:10 dilution in a Petri dish and a tube of lactose broth by following the directions given in Step 1. Label and incubate as stated in Step 1.	2.1. This technique makes a 1:10 dilution of the sample. 2.2. It is important that these measurements be as accurate as possible. 2.3. Use 1 ml of the 1:10 dilution in the Petri dish and the tube of lactose broth. 2.4. Be sure that the dilution is mixed thoroughly before transferring to the plate and the broth.

KEY STEPS

IMPORTANT POINTS

3. Prepare a 1:100 (1:H) dilution of the sample by transferring 9 ml of sterile distilled water to a sterile, dry test tube and adding 1 ml of the 1:10 dilution. Prepare cultures of the 1:H dilution by transferring 1 ml to a Petri dish and 1 ml with the same pipette to a tube of lactose broth. Label and incubate as stated in Step 1.

3.1. Again, make your measurements as accurate as possible.

4. Prepare a 1:1,000 (1:T) dilution using the same technique as given for preparing the 1:H dilution. Prepare cultures from the 1:T dilution as stated in Step 3.

4.1. These dilutions can be used as checks on each other when you count the plates.

Second Tests:
1. After a minimum of 24 hr but not more than 48 hr incubation at 37 C, prepare a plate of EMB agar for each sample of water used. Streak the EMB agar plate with a loopful of culture from the highest dilution of each sample in the lactose broth which has gas present in the fermentation tube. Label the plate and incubate at 37 C for 24 hr.

1.1. Spread the inoculum over the surface of the EMB agar so that you will have isolated colonies.
1.2. If more than 24 hr elapse between laboratory periods, place the plate in the refrigerator after the 24 hr of incubation.
1.3. A tube with any amount of gas is now considered positive; however, it used to be 10 per cent or more.

2. Count the number of colonies present on each plate prepared under "First Tests." Multiply by the dilution. Record the results.

2.1. Plates with less than 30 or more than 300 colonies *should not be counted.*
2.2. This gives the number of bacteria present per milliliter. What inaccuracies are there in this procedure?

Third Tests:
1. Select typical colonies from EMB agar prepared under "Second Tests." Inoculate material from each different kind of colony into separate tubes of lactose broth. Make nutrient agar slants from each kind of colony. Incubate the lactose broth and agar slant at 37 C.

1.1. *Escherichia coli* will produce dark purple colonies on EMB agar. These will appear to have a green metallic sheen. The colonies of *Enterobacter aerogenes* will be large raised colonies, rose-violet in color with little or no sheen. Other bacteria may grow on this medium at times, but most are inhibited.
1.2. Coliform organisms are gram-negative nonspore-forming rods that produce gas from lactose broth.

2. After incubation, make a Gram stain of the organisms on the nutrient agar slants. Record results. Look for gram-negative nonspore-forming rods.

Record of Observations:

1. Record the number of colonies in each plate. Record also the number of bacteria per milliliter.
2. Record the number of tubes showing any gas in lactose broth.
3. Record the results of the Gram stain.
4. Record the kind of colonies present on EMB agar medium.

RESULTS OF TESTS ON WATER
PLATE COUNT AND PRESUMPTIVE TEST

Sources of Samples of Water	Undiluted		1:10		1:H		1:T		Bacterial Count per Milliliter‡
	Lactose Broth*	Nutrient Agar† Plates	Lactose Broth	Nutrient Agar Plates	Lactose Broth	Nutrient Agar Plates	Lactose Broth	Nutrient Agar Plates	

*Record as "−", "+", or "⊕", for no acid, acid, or acid and gas production, respectively.

†Record as number of colonies counted.

‡Use exponents to report your results. Example: 184,000 is recorded as 1.8×10^5 MPN (most probable number) of cells per ml of original sample.

In many laboratories today coliform tests of water supplies are being conducted by the membrane filter (Millipore) method. Following is a summary of that method.

RESULTS OF TESTS ON WATER—CONTINUED.
MODIFIED CONFIRMED TEST AND COMPLETED TEST

Sources of Samples of Water	Undiluted		1:10		1:H		1:T	
	EMB Agar	Gram Stain	EMB Agar	Gram Stain	EMB Agar	Gram Stain	EMB Agar	Gram Stain

Questions:

1. Why is water tested only for intestinal organisms and not for pathogenic bacteria?

2. How do these organisms compare with those isolated from sewage?

3. Describe methods used by cities to insure safe water supply.

4. Name four diseases which might be transferred by means of water and state the etiology of each.

   a.

   b.

   c.

   d.

5. In order to prevent contamination of the water supply, what is the responsibility in caring for a patient who has typhoid fever?

6. Differentiate between "potable water" and "polluted water."

TOPIC: COLIFORM TEST ON WATER SUPPLIES BY THE MEMBRANE FILTER METHOD

EQUIPMENT:
1. Membrane filter assemblies (sterile).
2. Vacuum pump.
3. Side-arm vacuum flask (1,000 ml size) with hose.
4. Sterile graduates (100 ml size).
5. Sterile plastic Petri plates, 50 mm diameter.
6. Sterile membrane filter discs (Millipore #HAWG 047 AO).
7. Sterile water.
8. Sterile absorbent discs (packed with the membrane filters).
9. 5 ml pipettes.
10. 50 ml sterile M-HD Endo broth.
11. Water samples.
12. Forceps.
13. 70% ethanol.
14. Twelve 250 ml beakers.

Procedure:

1. Prepare a small plastic Petri plate (50 mm diameter) as follows:
   a. With sterile, flamed forceps, transfer aseptically a sterile absorbent pad to a sterile plastic Petri plate.
   b. With a 5 ml pipette transfer 1.8 to 2.0 ml M-HD Endo broth to the absorbent pad.
2. Assemble the membrane filtering unit by:
   a. Inserting the filter holder base into the neck of a one liter filter flask aseptically.
   b. With flamed forceps, place a sterile membrane filter disc aseptically, grid side up, on the filter holder base.
   c. Place the filter funnel on top of the membrane filter disc and secure it to the base with the clamp.
3. Vacuum filter the appropriate amount of water sample. Not less than 50 ml should be used. Waters of low turbidity and fewer bacteria permit samples of 200 ml or more.
4. Rinse the inner sides of the funnel with two 30 ml volumes of sterile water.
5. Remove the funnel and transfer aseptically the filter disc with sterile forceps to the Petri plate containing the absorbent pad moistened with the M-HD Endo broth. (Remember to keep the grid side up.)
6. Incubate the plate 18 to 24 hr at 35 C ± 0.5 C, without inverting the plate.
7. After suitable incubation, remove the filter from the plate and count the colonies on the disc with low power magnification, using reflected light. Disregard all colonies that lack the golden metallic sheen. The coliform density is reported in terms of coliforms per 100 ml of undiluted water sample.

Laboratory Exercise 30

TOPIC: BACTERIOLOGY OF MILK AND MILK PRODUCTS

OBJECTIVES: 1. To show the types and numbers of bacteria in milk.
2. To demonstrate the importance of pasteurization in milk.
3. To study microorganisms' survival in cold milk products.

EQUIPMENT: 1. Samples of raw and pasteurized milk (canned milk cannot be used).
2. Samples of ice cream, other milk derivatives, or sherbet.
3. Sterile 1 ml pipettes.
4. Sterile 10 ml pipettes.
5. Sterile distilled water.
6. Sterile test tubes.
7. Sterile Petri dishes.
8. Sterile heart infusion agar for plating.

Procedure:

KEY STEPS	IMPORTANT POINTS
1. Prepare the following dilutions of the milk samples: 1:H; 1:T; 1:10T; 1:HT.	1.1. Use the same technique that is described in Exercise 29. 1.2. How would you make a 1:T dilution using the bottle dilution method? See the drawings of the dilution scheme after Exercise 28.
2. Prepare pour plates of the dilutions.	2.1. Why do you not use the 1:10 dilution?
3. If you are testing raw milk, do not plate the 1: H dilution.	3.1. Why?
4. Allow the heart infusion agar to harden, label, invert and incubate the plates at 37 C for 48 hr. Count the colonies.	4.1. Count the colonies on plates that have more than 30 but less than 300 colonies. See the instructions on counting colonies after Exercise 28.
5. Repeat the procedures as given in Steps 1, 3, and 4 for a sample of ice cream. Start out with an 1 g of ice cream in 99 ml sterile water (1:H dilution).	5.1. Do you expect bacteria in ice cream?

Record of Observations:

1. Record all results in the chart provided and multiply by the dilution.

RESULTS OF TESTS IN MILK AND MILK PRODUCTS

Dilutions	Raw Milk*		Pasteurized Milk		Ice Cream	
	No. of Colonies per Plate	Bacteria per ml of undiluted milk	No. of Colonies per plate	Bacteria per ml of undiluted milk	No. of Colonies per plate	Bacteria per ml of undiluted ice cream
1:H	✕	✕				
1:T						
1:10T						
1:HT						
Average count per ml	✕		✕		✕	

*Use exponents to record your results (see Exercise 29).

Questions:

1. Why did you use higher dilutions of raw milk than for pasteurized milk?

2. What are the sources of bacteria in milk?

3. What is meant by certified milk?

4. What diseases may be transferred by milk and what is the etiology of each?

5. What other types of milk are commonly used today? Why are these products not suitable for this experiment?

6. What other milk products could we have tested? With what possible results?

7. Would you expect microorganisms on cheeses? If so, why?

Laboratory Exercise 31

TOPIC: METHODS USED IN MYCOLOGY

OBJECTIVES: 1. To make the student aware of the importance of mycology.
2. To learn simple techniques used to differentiate species of molds, pathogens and nonpathogens.

EQUIPMENT: 1. A culture of *Penicillium.*
2. A culture of *Aspergillus.*
3. Some moldy bread, fruit, lemon, etc.
4. Sabouraud's Glucose Agar in Petri plates.
5. Lactophenol cotton blue stain.
6. Petri dishes, sterile.
7. Short glass rods.
8. Filter paper soaked in 50 per cent glycerol.
9. Glass slides and coverslips.

Procedure:

Medium used: ***Sabouraud's Glucose Agar*** (commercially available)

Glucose	40 g
Agar	35 g
Peptone	10 g
Distilled water	1,000 ml

pH adjusted to 5.5

Antibiotics may be added to cool—but not solid—medium to discourage bacterial growth, but they are not really necessary.

Lactophenol cotton blue stain (for fungal cultures)—also known as ***Linder's Solution***

Lactic acid	20 ml
Phenol	20 g
Glycerol	40 ml
Distilled water	20 ml

After the mixture is slightly heated in hot water, 0.05 g cotton blue (or aniline blue) is added. Fungal structures stain deep blue, and the background is pale blue. See Step 5.

The slide culture technique

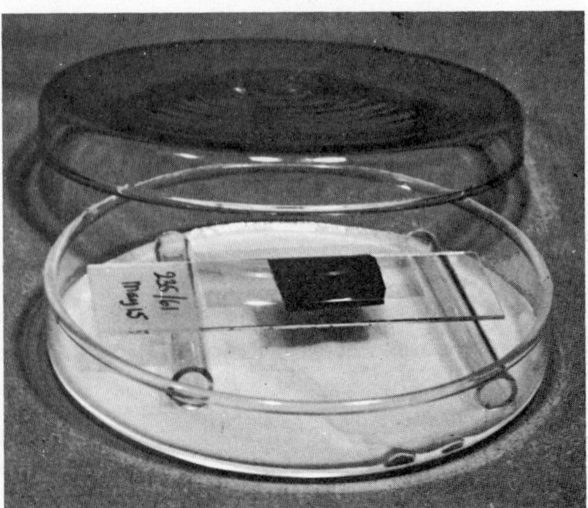

The details of the technique are given in Step 2.

The giant colony technique

(Illustrations from Conant et al.:*Manual of Clinical Mycology.* 3rd Ed. Philadelphia, W. B. Saunders Co., 1971.)

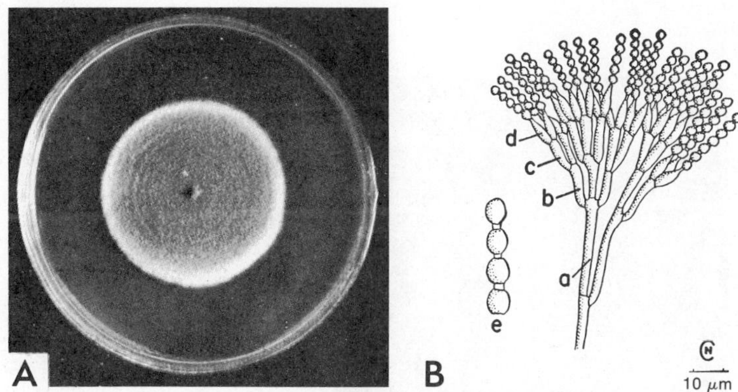

Penicillium sp.

A, Penicillium sp. The rapidly growing colony (50 mm in diameter, 8 days) is at first white, then becomes bluish-green and very powdery due to abundant spore production from the aerial mycelium.

B, Penicillium sp. Spore-bearing hyphae characteristically form a "penicillus," or brush. The conidia occur in unbranched chains (e) cut off from the tip of flask-shaped sterigmata (d) which are verticillately arranged (in whorls) from the ends of metulae (c) arising from branches (b) of the conidiophore (a).

Although species of *Penicillium* differ in gross appearance (size of colony, color, texture, etc.), the genus may be identified by the characteristic structure of the conidiophore which arises from vegetative hyphae in, on or above the agar, at the end of which branching takes place to form the typical "penicillus," or brush.

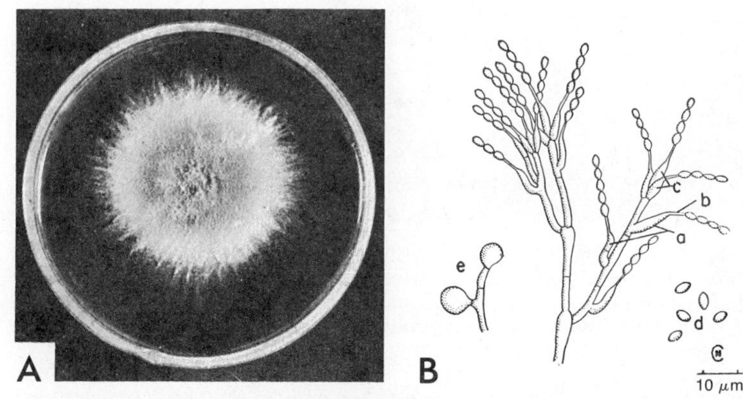

Paecilomyces sp.

A, Paecilomyces sp. The rapidly growing colony (70 mm in diameter, 5 days) thinly covers the agar surface and becomes yellowish-brown and powdery due to an abundant production of conidia.

B, Paecilomyces sp. The conidial-bearing hyphae superficially resemble the "penicillus" of *Penicillium.* Elliptical conidia (d) occur in unbranched chains cut off from the tip of flask-shaped sterigmata (c) which not only appear verticillately arranged (in whorls) on the ends of hyphae, but a single sterigma may also appear along a hypha (a). The appearance of the single sterigma (a) from the hypha and its characteristic taper into a long, conidial-bearing tube (b) which bends away from the main axis of the sterigma, and the accessory cells or "macrospores" (e) found in or close to the surface of the agar, distinguish this fungus from those of the genus *Penicillium.*

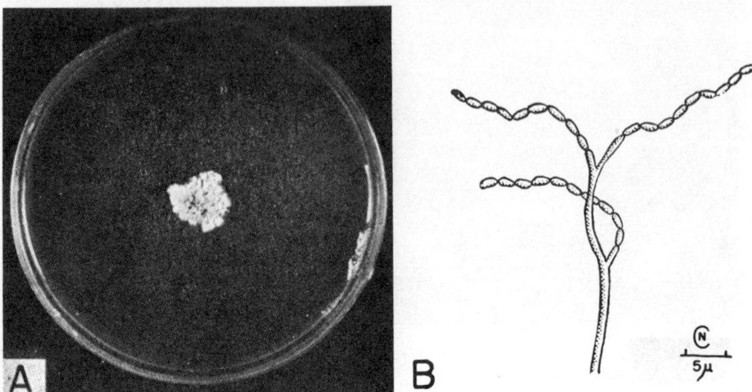

A, *Streptomyces (Actinomyces)* sp. The slow-growing, leathery colony (17 mm in diameter, 26 days) becomes somewhat wrinkled, covered with a fine, chalky white surface, and has a distinct, pungent, musty odor. Many species produce a variety of colors due to characteristic pigment formation.

B, *Streptomyces (Actinomyces)* sp. Long, slender, branching hyphae (1 μm in diameter) produce spores by fragmentation or segmentation of the terminal branches. Microscopic preparations are not made easily, and it is usually necessary to study the morphology of the fungi from slide cultures. These saprophytic organisms occur commonly in the soil and are frequent contaminants in the laboratory.

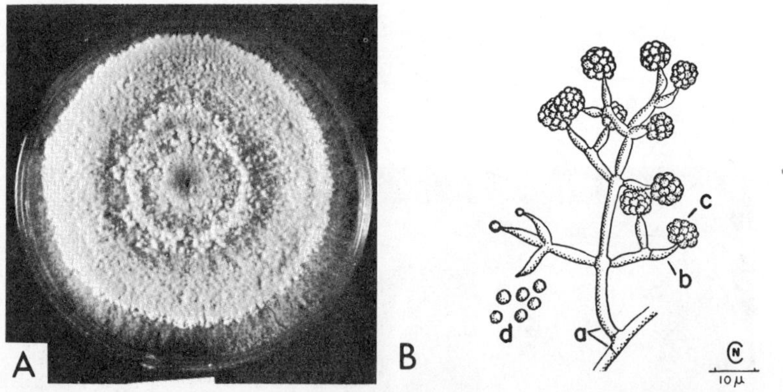

A, *Trichoderma* sp. The rapidly growing colony fills the petri dish in 5 days with a thin growth over the surface of the agar. Compact, woolly tufts of white mycelium appear gradually, forming a dense mat which becomes green with the production of conidia. Test tube cultures macroscopically simulate species of *Penicillium* in color, but the prolific growth and microscopic morphology readily distinguish these forms.

B, *Trichoderma* sp. The conidiophores (b) are short, irregular branches from the vegetative mycelium (a) and are not arranged in whorls. Spherical, single-celled conidia (d) form globular clusters at the ends of these conidiophores (c) but are dissociated easily. They are not readily seen unless microscopic preparations are made with great care.

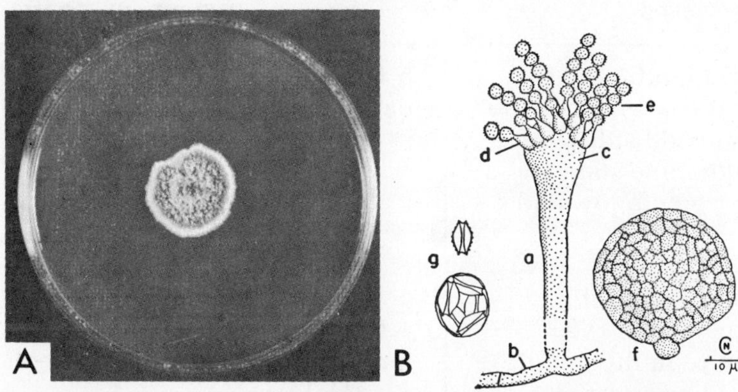

A, Aspergillus sp. The compact, slow-growing colony (28 mm in diameter, 8 days) is at first white, then becomes bluish-green with sulfur-yellow areas scattered over the surface.

B, Aspergillus sp. The conidial-bearing structure is an unbranched, nonseptate, elongate hypha (a) arising from a foot cell (b) in the mycelium. It is enlarged at the tip, forming a vesicle (c) from which flask-shaped sterigmata (d) are produced which completely or partially cover the swollen surface. Conidia are cut off from the tips of the sterigmata, forming unbranched chains (e) and giving a rough appearance to the apically swollen conidiophore. Some species of *Aspergillus* develop perithecia (f) containing asci and ascospores (g). When these structures are encountered, the fungus is placed among the Ascomycetes in the genus *Eurotium*.

KEY STEPS	IMPORTANT POINTS
The Growth of Molds 1. Look at the results obtained and drawings made in Exercise 3.	1.1. Would it have helped to stain the fungal structures you drew in Exercise 3?
2. Prepare a Petri plate with two glass rods on filter paper soaked in 50 per cent glycerol. See the photograph on page 140.	2.1. The filter paper is kept wet so that culture does not dry out. Why use glycerol?
3. Put a piece of Sabouraud's Glucose Agar on a glass slide, put mold spores on the medium and sandwich it between the slide and a coverslip on top. Put the slide over the rods in the Petri dish and incubate for several days.	3.1. This type of culture technique was developed from an earlier used method, called the Henrici Slide Culture. 3.2. Note that fungal cultures are very slow to grow. 3.3. When do the spores begin to form from the mycelium?
4. During the incubation period observe the growth of the mold and the development of spores microscopically, using low illumination.	

KEY STEPS	**IMPORTANT POINTS**

5. Pick up a small portion of the fungal colony with a sterile needle, put on a slide and add a drop of lactophenol cotton blue stain and a coverslip. Observe with low and high power.

5.1. Remember that fungal structures stain dark blue, the background pale blue.

The Giant Colony Technique

1. Put a small amount of the *Penicillium* culture in the middle of a Sabouraud's Glucose Agar Petri plate. Incubate for several days.

1.1. Sabouraud's Glucose Agar is an excellent medium for the growth of molds. Its low pH inhibits bacteria.

1.2. Other media that can be used are Mycological Agar, Mycophil Agar, Phyton Yeast Extract Agar, Mycosel Agar, Dermatophyte Test Medium (DTM), Corn Meal Agar, and others.

2. Do the same with *Aspergillus* and some other mold from the fruit, bread, or other food. Label all plates.

2.1. Would *Aspergillus* form different giant colonies than *Penicillium?* Why?

3. Note the formation differences of the giant colonies and compare with the illustrations shown on pages 141 to 143.

3.1. Note the undisturbed spore formation on the giant plates.

3.2. Do not open any of these plates but autoclave them well. You do not wish to contaminate the entire laboratory with mold spores.

Questions:

1. Why is it important to recognize fungal species?

2. What is a dermatomycosis?

3. What is a superficial mycosis?

4. Name some systemic or deep mycoses.

Laboratory Exercise 32

TOPIC: IMMUNIZING AGENTS

OBJECTIVES: 1. To demonstrate the available immunizing agents.
2. To familiarize the student with the use of different immunizing agents.

EQUIPMENT: 1. Samples of as many vaccines, toxoids, antisera and antitoxins as possible, manufacturers' instruction for handling and use.

Procedure:

KEY STEPS	IMPORTANT POINTS
1. Examine all of the samples of immunizing agents provided.	1.1. Differentiate between those which contain antigens and those which contain antibodies.
2. Study the manufacturers' instructions for handling and use.	2.1. How are these instructions similar? 2.2. What differences are there?

Record of Observations:

1. Fill in the chart on immunizing agents.

Questions:

1. Define:

 a. Antigen

 b. Antibody

 c. Vaccine

 d. Toxoid

 e. Antiserum

 f. Antitoxin

2. What immunizing agents are recommended for use from age 6 months to 5 years. Why?

3. What is a "booster dose"? Why is it used?

4. When would antisera and antitoxins be used? Why?

5. Differentiate between antisera and antitoxins.

6. What immunizing agents should be readministered periodically during life? Why?

7. What immunizing agent may still be readministered periodically during life, but is now considered elective. Why?

8. What immunizations are recommended prior to travel outside the United States? Why?

PREVENTIVE VACCINES AGAINST INFECTIOUS DISEASES OF HUMANS

PRACTICAL SCHEDULE FOR ACTIVE IMMUNIZATION IN CHILDREN

Age	Vaccine (Immunogen)	Diseases
2–3 Months	DTP (Toxoids of diphtheria and tetanus, and pertussis [whooping cough] bacterial antigen)	Diphtheria Tetanus Pertussis
	Oral active (Sabin) trivalent poliovaccine	Poliomyelitis
4–5 Months	DTP	
6–7 Months	DTP Poliovaccine, oral trivalent	
12 Months	Measles, attenuated vaccine (Edmonston strain given with gamma globulins; Schwarz strain, without)	Rubeola
15–19 Months	Smallpox vaccine (active vaccinia virus)—elective DTP Poliovaccine, oral trivalent	Smallpox
1–2 Years*	Mumps vaccine (active, attenuated)	Mumps
4–6 Years*	DTP Smallpox vaccine—elective Poliovaccine, oral trivalent	
1–10 Years*	Rubella vaccine (active, attentuated)	Rubella
12–14 Years*	TD (tetanus toxoid and diphtheria toxoid; adult type) Smallpox vaccine—elective	

PREVENTION OF DISEASES NOT INCLUDED IN THE ABOVE SCHEDULE

	Active virus (attenuated)	Yellow fever
	Inactivated virus	Rabies, influenza
	Killed *Rickettsia prowazekii*	Typhus fever
These vaccines may be given electively wherever indicated	Killed bacteria (*Salmonella typhi, S. paratyphi S. schottmuelleri*)	Typhoid fever and paratyphoid fever
	Purified polysaccharide of *Streptococcus pneumoniae*	Pneumonia
	Purified polysaccharide of *Neisseria meningitidis* (groups A and C)	Cerebrospinal meningitis
	Cell extract of *Vibrio cholerae*	Cholera
	Cell extract of *Yersinia pestis*	Plague
	Infectious attenuated mycobacteria (*BCG, Bacille Calmette Guérin*)	Tuberculosis

*A tuberculin test may be administered in high risk populations.

It is hoped that vaccines against infectious and serum hepatitis and herpes virus-caused diseases will soon be added to the above list.

CHART OF IMMUNIZING AGENTS

Immunizing Agent	Protection Against What Disease?	Duration of Protection	When Administered	How Administered	Dosage	Reaction (If Any)
A. Antigens:						
1. Typhoid vaccine						
2. Paratyphoid vaccine						
3. Diphtheria toxoid						
4. Tetanus toxoid						
5. Smallpox vaccine						
6. Pertussis vaccine						
7. BCG						
8. Salk vaccine						
9. Influenza vaccine						
10. Sabin vaccine						
11. Rubella vaccine						
12. Rubeola vaccine						
B. Antibodies:						
1. Diphtheria antitoxin						
2. Tetanus antitoxin						
3. Meningococcus antiserum						
4. Antistreptococcus serum						
5. Botulism antitoxin						
6. Gas gangrene antitoxin						
7. Gamma globulin						
8.						
9.						

Laboratory Exercise 33

TOPIC: BIOLOGICAL SUBSTANCES USED FOR TESTING

OBJECTIVES: 1. To show some substances used for testing susceptibility to infection.
2. To show some substances used for diagnostic purposes.

EQUIPMENT: 1. Materials for the Dick test.
2. Materials for the Schick test.
3. Materials for the tuberculin test.
4. Materials used in testing for allergies.

Procedure:

KEY STEPS	IMPORTANT POINTS
1. Examine materials used for the Dick, Schick, the tuberculin and the allergy tests.	1.1. How are the Dick and Schick tests similar?
2. Study the instructions given by the manufacturers for use and handling of these materials.	2.1. What are the similarities and differences between the tuberculin test and allergy tests?

Record of Observations:

1. Record the information as listed on the table provided on the next page.

Questions:

1. Define:

   a. Toxin

   b. Tuberculin

   c. Allergen

2. Discuss the advantages and disadvantages of the Dick test, the Schick test and the tuberculin test.

3. What is the purpose of the control in the Schick and Dick tests?

4. What is the relationship of the tests for allergies to immunity?

BIOLOGICAL TESTS AND ALLERGENS

Tests	When Used	Purpose	Interpretation of Results	
			Positive	Negative
Dick test				
Schick test				
Tuberculin test				
Allergens, pollen: 1.				
2.				
3.				
4.				
5.				
Allergens, food: 1.				
2.				
3.				
4.				
5.				
Allergens, other: 1.				
2.				
3.				
4.				
5.				

On the following pages there is reproduced a tabulation of scratch tests employed at an actual allergy clinic, demonstrating the wide range of substances that can act as allergens.

Allergy Clinic

SCRATCH TESTS

PATIENT_______________________________   DATE__________________

POLLENS

1. Control ____	19. Sweet Gum ____	37. Red Top ____
2. Fall (Cedar) Elm ____	20. Mimosa ____	38. Sudan ____
3. Mt. Cedar ____	21. Narrow Marshelder ____	39. Sweet Vernal ____
4. Red Cedar ____	22. Rough Marshelder ____	40. Orchard Grass ____
5. Black Willow ____	23. Cocklebur ____	41. Russian Thistle ____
6. Black Walnut ____	24. Short Ragweed ____	42. Lamb's Quarter ____
7. Box Elder ____	25. Giant Ragweed ____	43. Shad Scale ____
8. Hickory ____	26. False Ragweed ____	44. Kochia ____
9. Pecan ____	27. Western Ragweed ____	45. Common Wormwood ____
10. Elm ____	28. Johnson Grass ____	46. Sagebrush ____
11. Cottonwood ____	29. Johnson Grass Smut ____	47. West. Water Hemp. ____
12. Mesquite ____	30. Annual Bluegrass ____	48. Spiney Amaranth ____
13. Sycamore ____	31. Perennial Rye Grass ____	49. Palmer's Amaranth ____
14. Pine ____	32. Bermuda Grass ____	50. Privet ____
15. Hackberry ____	33. Bermuda Grass Smut ____	51. English Plantain ____
16. Green Ash ____	34. Salt Grass ____	52. Sunflower ____
17. Oak ____	35. Timothy ____	53. Rose ____
18. River Birch ____	36. Smooth Brome ____	54. Chrysanthemum ____

MOLDS & EPIDERMALS

1. House Dust ____	15. Cattle Hair ____	29. Rayon ____
2. Monilia ____	16. Horse Hair ____	30. Cottonseed ____
3. Helminthosporium ____	17. Dog ____	31. Cotton Linters ____
4. Hormodendrum ____	18. Cat ____	32. Jute ____
5. Alternaria ____	19. Sheep Wool ____	33. Hemp ____
6. Aspergillus ____	20. Orris Root ____	34. Glue ____
7. Chaetomium ____	21. Kapok ____	35. Gum Tragacanth ____
8. Rhizopus ____	22. Pyrethrum ____	36. Gum Acacia ____
9. Penicillium ____	23. Tobacco ____	37. Gum Kayara ____
10. Mucor ____	24. Cigar Smoke ____	38. ____
11. Trichophyton ____	25. Rabbit ____	39. ____
12. Duck Feathers ____	26. Camel Hair ____	40. ____
13. Chicken Feathers ____	27. Silk ____	41. ____
14. Parakeet Feathers ____	28. Flaxseed ____	42. ____

Table continued on the following page

SCRATCH TESTS (*Continued*)

FOODS

Legumes		Vegetables		Fruits		Seafood	
1. Lima Bean	____	25. Celery	____	50. Avocado	____	75. Tuna	____
2. Navy Bean	____	26. Onion	____	51. Banana	____	76. Salmon	____
3. Soy Bean	____	27. Garlic	____	52. Coconut	____	77. Shrimp	____
4. Green Bean	____	28. Green Pepper	____	53. Strawberry	____	78. Lobster	____
5. Blackeye Pea	____	29. White Potato	____	54. Blackberry	____	79. Oyster	____
6. Green Pea	____	30. Sweet Potato	____	55. Cranberry	____	80. Haddock	____
7. Almond	____	31. Spinach	____	56. Raspberry	____	81. Flounder	____
8. Peanut	____	32. Mustard Greens	____	57. Lemon	____	82. Catfish	____
9. Pecan	____	33. Lettuce	____	58. Lime	____	83. Trout	____
10. English Walnut	____	34. Asparagus	____	59. Grapefruit	____	84. Bass	____
		35. Broccoli	____	60. Orange	____	85. Perch	____
Cereal Grains		36. Brussels Sprouts	____	61. Pineapple	____		
11. Corn	____	37. Cabbage	____	62. Peach	____	Spice	
12. Barley	____	38. Cauliflower	____	63. Pear	____	86. Mustard	____
13. Buckwheat	____	39. Beets	____	64. Plum	____	87. Allspice	____
14. Oats	____	40. Turnip	____	65. Cherry	____	88. Black Pepper	____
15. Rice	____	41. Carrot	____	66. Apple	____	89. Chili Pepper	____
16. Rye	____	42. Radish	____	67. Cantaloupe	____	90. Cinnamon	____
17. Wheat	____	43. Squash	____	68. Grape	____	91. Cloves	____
		44. Cucumber	____	69. Olive	____	92. Dill	____
Milk		45. Mushroom	____	70. Watermelon	____	93. Nutmeg	____
18. Cow Casein	____	46. Tomato	____			94. Vanilla	____
19. Cow Whey	____			Beverages		95. Sage	____
		Meats		71. Chocolate	____		
Egg		47. Beef	____	72. Coffee	____	Misc.	
20. Egg White	____	48. Lamb	____	73. Tea	____	96. Baker's Yeast	____
21. Egg Yolk	____	49. Pork	____	74. Peppermint	____	97. Brewer's Yeast	____
						98. Hops	____
Fowl						99. Malt	____
22. Chicken	____					100. Cola	____
23. Duck	____						
24. Turkey	____						

±indicates a slight, or questionable reaction.

Laboratory Exercise 34

TOPIC: BLOOD TYPING

OBJECTIVE: 1. To help students understand the bases of blood typing and reactions to blood transfusions.

EQUIPMENT: 1. Commercial anti-A serum and anti-B serum.
2. Clean microscope slides.
3. 70 per cent ethyl alcohol.
4. Sterile cotton balls or gauze squares.
5. Sterile blood lancets.
6. Toothpicks.

Procedure:

KEY STEPS	IMPORTANT POINTS
1. Draw a line longitudinally across the center of a microscope slide.	
2. Mark half of the slide "Anti-A" and the other half "Anti-B."	
3. Place one drop of anti-A serum on the half of the slide marked "Anti-A."	3.1. *Precaution:* Do not use the same dropper for anti-A and anti-B serum. Why?
4. Repeat Step 3 using anti-B serum.	
5. Clean the tip of your index finger thoroughly with sterile cotton balls or gauze squares moistened with 70 per cent ethyl alcohol. Small packages for this purpose are also commercially available. *Note:* It may be easier to work in pairs on this step.	5.1. Why should you clean the skin thoroughly with 70 per cent ethyl alcohol?
6. Puncture the tip of the index finger deeply enough to release several drops of blood. Use a prepackaged sterile lancet or hemolet. *Never* use the old-fashioned automatic instrument that punctured the finger, was sterilized and used again, etc.	6.1. It is less painful to stick the finger once well, and without hesitation. 6.2. Why would an automatic puncturing device, that was sterilized between uses, be less desirable than a disposable lancet?
7. Place one drop of blood next to the anti-A serum and another drop of blood adjacent to the anti-B serum.	

KEY STEPS	IMPORTANT POINTS

8. Mix the drop of blood and serum on each half of the slide with the clean toothpick, using one end for one serum and the other end for the second serum.

8.1. Why must a separate *end* of the toothpick be used for each type of serum?

9. Tilt the slide but avoid mixing the drops from both sides.

9.1. Why should the slide be tilted?

9.2. Why should you avoid mixing?

10. Observe any agglutination with the naked eye and with the low and high power magnification of the microscope. Continue the observation for 5 min before discarding the slide.

10.1. Why are microscopic examinations essential?

10.2. Why must a time interval of 5 min be allowed before discarding?

Record of Results:

1. Record the results of all members of your laboratory section on the next page according to the following scheme:

BLOOD GROUP TESTING REACTION SCHEME

Reactions with Sera		Blood Group Being Tested Is
Anti-A	Anti-B	
−	−	O
+	−	A
−	+	B
+	+	AB

− = no agglutination; + = agglutination

Caution: Because of the possibility that the sera you used were "expired sera" that may have to be used up, *do not depend on your blood type to be accurate* and do not base any reliability on these blood tests. The clinical laboratory would normally use sera much more quickly than some teaching laboratories, therefore it is expected to have fresh, more reliable sera on hand to use for blood testing, etc.

Name of Student	Number in Each Major Blood Grouping			
	O	A	B	AB
1.				
2.				
3.				
4.				
5.				
6.				
7.				
8.				
9.				
10.				
11.				
12.				
13.				
14.				
15.				

Questions:

1. What are the national percentages for each of the major blood groups?

   O___________%; A___________%; B___________%; AB___________%.

2. What is the basis for this agglutination phenomenon?

3. What are agglutinogens?

4. What are some of the causes of reactions to blood transfusions?

5. Identify factors other than those responsible for the major blood groups which may result in antigen-antibody reaction causing either agglutination or hemolysis. What is the importance of these other factors?

Laboratory Exercise 35

TOPIC: PRECIPITIN TEST

OBJECTIVE: 1. To become familiar with a test that has many practical applications in medical-legal work, also in the food industry and in testing of antibody production by animals.

EQUIPMENT:
1. Human serum.
2. Anti-human serum (horse or rabbit serum).
3. Human blood and lancets.
4. Rabbit serum.
5. Anti-rabbit serum (probably from horse).
6. Linen or other material.
7. Disposable micropipettes (Pasteur pipettes) and bulbs.
8. Small precipitin test tubes.
9. 1 ml pipettes.
10. Test tubes for dilutions.
11. Saline solution.

Procedure: Each student will perform *one* precipitin test using *one* of the following:

1. Human serum and anti-human serum.
2. Human blood and anti-human serum.
3. Rabbit serum and anti-rabbit serum.

No sterile techniques are needed or required.

KEY STEPS	**IMPORTANT POINTS**
1. A small piece of linen is spotted with serum or a student's blood. A spotted area of the linen is soaked in 1 ml saline. A nonspotted piece of the same linen is also soaked in 1 ml saline.	1.1. Which linen piece is the antigen containing sample? 1.2. Why is a linen control necessary?
2. The test is performed by pipetting the antiserum to 8 small test tubes. The antibody dilutions are then gently layered above the antiserum with a Pasteur pipette, by pulling the pipette slowly up the inside wall of the tube and depressing the rubber bulb.	2.1. Why should the test tubes be as small as possible? 2.2. Note that the two layers of antiserum (bottom) and antigen (top) do not mix. Why? 2.3. Your technique requires only caution and a steady hand.
3. Note the test scheme for all 8 tubes as shown following Step 4.	

KEY STEPS	**IMPORTANT POINTS**
4. Examine all tubes for precipitation at the interphase of the two liquids after 30 min and 1 hr. Keep at room temperature. If there are no results, examine after 2 hr.	4.1. You have to hold the tube against the light and observe it carefully. Compare with the control tubes. 4.2. This test can also be performed on a plate. 4.3. What is the Ouchterlony plate technique?

TEST SCHEME

Tube number	Lower layer	Upper layer	Expected results
1	Antiserum	Spot extract	
2	Antiserum	Spot extract 1:10	
3	Antiserum	Spot extract 1:H	
4 Control	Antiserum	Known serum	Precipitation
5 Control	Antiserum	Heterologous serum	No precipitation
6 Control	Antiserum	Linen extract	No precipitation
7 Control	Antiserum	Saline	No precipitation
8 Control	Normal rabbit serum or proper control serum	Spot extract	No precipitation

Record of Observations:

1. Report the titer and your interpretation of the test.

Questions:

1. What was the titer?

2. What did your test indicate?

3. Name two tests in medicine that are precipitin tests.

   a.

   b.

Laboratory Exercise 36

TOPIC: KOLMER-WASSERMANN TEST (COMPLEMENT FIXATION) DEMONSTRATION

OBJECTIVES:
1. To demonstrate the function of complement.
2. To show an historically very important test.
3. To demonstrate to the student the complexity of serological tests.
4. To discuss diagnosis of syphilis and BFP (biologically false positive) reactions.

EQUIPMENT:
1. BBL (formally Baltimore Biological Laboratory) kit for the Kolmer-Wassermann test.
2. Pipettes.
3. Test tubes.

Procedure: For your information an exact procedure for the test with the BBL (Baltimore Biological Laboratory) kit is reproduced here from the instructions in the kit. The instructor and student should not expect every kit to contain the same identical instructions; therefore, the directions given here should only be considered as sample directions. Follow the exact procedure given in *your* Kolmer-Wassermann test kit.

POSITIVE SYPHILITIC SERUM, BBL PREPARATION

BBL Positive Syphilitic Serum has been carefully prepared and standardized so that, when restored according to directions, it will react in accordance with the table shown on page 152.

RESTORATION OF THE LYOPHILIZED, POSITIVE SYPHILITIC SERUM

1. Remove the stopper from the vial, being careful to prevent particles of the lyophilized material from adhering to the stopper.
2. Using a 5 ml pipette, point to point, pipette the appropriate amount of distilled water into the vial (1 ml in the 1 ml vial or 3 ml in the 3 ml vial).
3. Replace the stopper and agitate gently until all of the material is dissolved.
4. The reconstituted material represents undiluted serum. Whole serum or dilutions should be heated for 30 min at 56 C, before use.

STORAGE

1. Unopened vials should be stored at temperatures below 5 C.
2. The reconstituted control serum may be tested over a period of *not more than 5 days,* if desired, by pipetting aliquots of each dilution into individual tubes, tightly stoppering, and preserving by storage in the frozen state. (Do not store in dry ice.)

TABLE OF DILUTIONS

Full Volume Kolmer-Wassermann

Tube	Serum (ml)	Saline (ml)	Dilution	Reaction
1	1.0 undiluted	7.0	1/8	No hemolysis
2	1.0 of tube 1	1.0	1/16	50% partial hemolysis (3+)
3	1.0 of tube 2	1.0	1/32	Complete hemolysis

Preparation of test constituents:

BALANCED KIT FOR KOLMER-WASSERMANN TEST FOR 25 TESTS

Reagent	Volume	Physical State	Container	Restore With	Volume Used Per Test
Kolmer-Wassermann antigen (cardiolipin)	0.1 ml	In alcohol	20 ml sealed glass ampul	15 ml of saline	0.5 ml
Pooled guinea pig complement	1.2 ml Titer: 1/50	Desiccated	60 ml serum vial	60 ml of saline	2.0 ml
Anti-sheep hemolysin	1 ml of 1/100 dilution Titer: 1/6,000	In 50% Glycerin	30 ml serum vial	29 ml of saline	1.0 ml
Physiological saline	8 oz	Fluid	8 oz bottle		
Washed sheep cells (10% suspension)	6 ml	Fluid	30 ml bottle	24 ml of saline	1.0 ml
Positive syphilitic serum (4 plus)	1 ml	Desiccated	Sealed tube	1 ml of distilled water	

Store at room temperature:
Kolmer-Wassermann cardiolipin antigen
Physiologic saline

Store in refrigerator:
Pooled guinea pig complement
Anti-sheep hemolysin
Washed, pooled sheep cells,
  10% suspension
Positive control sera

Test scheme:

Add Amounts Indicated in Order Listed	Tube 1	Tube 2	Antigen Control	Hemolytic System Control	Control
Serum to be tested	0.2 ml	0.2 ml	- - - -	- - - -	- - - -
Kolmer-Wassermann Cardiolipin antigen	0.5 ml	- - - -	0.5 ml	- - - -	- - - -
Complement	1.0 ml	1.0 ml	1.0 ml	1.0 ml	- - - -
Saline	0.3 ml	0.8 ml	0.5 ml	1.0 ml	2.5 ml

INCUBATE OVERNIGHT IN REFRIGERATOR

Anti-Sheep Hemolysin	0.5 ml	0.5 ml	0.5 ml	0.5 ml	- - - -
Sheep cells 2%	0.5 ml	0.5 ml	0.5 ml	0.5 ml	0.5 ml

INCUBATE AT 37 C

10 min after Tube 2 shows sparking hemolysis, make reading on Tube 1. Antigen control may take 60 min to show complete hemolysis.

READ AS FOLLOWS (REFERENCE IS TO AMOUNT OF HEMOLYSIS IN TUBES):

4 plus reading	None	Complete	Complete	Complete	None
2 plus reading	Partial	Complete	Complete	Complete	None
Negative reading	Complete	Complete	Complete	Complete	None

Try to understand this test and the results obtained. Follow the directions of your instructor to report your results.

Laboratory Exercise 37

TOPIC: ANAPHYLACTIC SHOCK (DEMONSTRATION)

OBJECTIVE: 1. To demonstrate anaphylaxis in a guinea pig.

EQUIPMENT: 1. Two guinea pigs.
2. Sterile horse serum (any antitoxin or antiserum can be substituted if it has been prepared in horses).
3. Sterile 2 ml syringe and needle.
4. Dissecting kit.

Procedure:

KEY STEPS	IMPORTANT POINTS
1. Ten to 14 days prior to this demonstration your instructor will have you inject one guinea pig with 2 ml of sterile horse serum. Mark this animal so that you can identify it.	1.1. Why is this time period essential?
2. Ten to 14 days later inject both guinea pigs with 0.5 ml of sterile horse serum and have the class observe the results.	2.1. What happened? 2.2. Why did it happen?
3. After the test guinea pig is dead, autopsy it and have the class observe the internal organs.	3.1. What did you observe?

Record of Observations:

1. See "Important Points."

Questions:

1. What is anaphylaxis?

What is serum sickness?

What is allergy?

2. What kinds of substances can produce allergic reactions?

3. What is the present explanation for this phenomenon?

PATHOGENIC MICROORGANISMS

The purpose of this unit is to introduce students to the field of pathogenic micro-organisms so that they can recognize the importance of this group of organisms, begin to build a background of information for clinical applications, and correlate and co-ordinate information and knowledge of the preceding units into a better understanding of the relationship of microbiology to the practice of medical science. It is advisable and desirable for the students to prepare their own charts from reference sources rather than copy any information from charts which have been published. The more time and effort each student puts into the development of this correlated information, the better will be the understanding of this material. Only those aspects of the medical field that have a direct relation to microbiology will be considered.

Because hospital personnel have a primary responsibility in preventing transfer of pathogenic microorganisms, the charts have been arranged according to the following categories: pathogens transmitted from the intestinal and/or urinary tract, pathogens transmitted from the respiratory tract, pathogens transmitted from the genital tract, pathogens from the soil, and blood-borne infections. If a particular course in microbiology is being taught according to morphologic characteristics of pathogens, it will be possible to use this section because each chart has been arranged according to the following sequence: pathogenic cocci, gram-negative bacilli, gram-positive bacilli, spiro-chetes, rickettsias, viruses, pathogenic fungi, and protozoa. This arrangement permits the assignment of sections from different charts to be completed with a group of micro-organisms having like morphologic characteristics.

A. PATHOGENS TRANSMITTED FROM THE INTESTINAL AND/OR URINARY TRACT

Laboratory Exercise 38

TOPIC: PATHOGENIC MICROORGANISMS OF THE INTESTINAL AND URINARY TRACTS

OBJECTIVES: 1. To understand the characteristics of the pathogenic members of the enteric group of bacteria.
2. To understand the characteristics of the enteric group of viruses and protozoa.
3. To relate these organisms to certain diseases.

EQUIPMENT:* 1. Prepared slides of species of *Salmonella* and *Shigella* or 35 mm slides for projection.
2. 24 hr broth culture of *Salmonella typhi.*
3. Serum containing H-agglutinins for *S. typhi.*
4. Sterile saline solution.

Procedure:

KEY STEPS	IMPORTANT POINTS
1. Prepare two hanging drop slides of **S. *typhi.***	1.1. This is a pathogenic organism. 1.2. The instructor may prefer to set this up as a demonstration.
2. To one drop add a drop of anti-typhoid serum. To the second drop add a drop of sterile saline.	2.1. What is the name of this test? 2.2. When would this test be used?
3. Examine boths slides with the high dry power of the microscope.	
4. Examine slides of **Salmonella** and **Shigella.**	

---

*As a component of this exercise the instructor may choose to demonstrate the use of the Enterotube (Hoffmann-LaRoche, Inc.), which provides a means for rapid differential identification of gram-negative bacteria *(Enterobacteriaceae).*

Record of Observations:

1. Record observations from a hanging drop of *Salmonella typhi.*

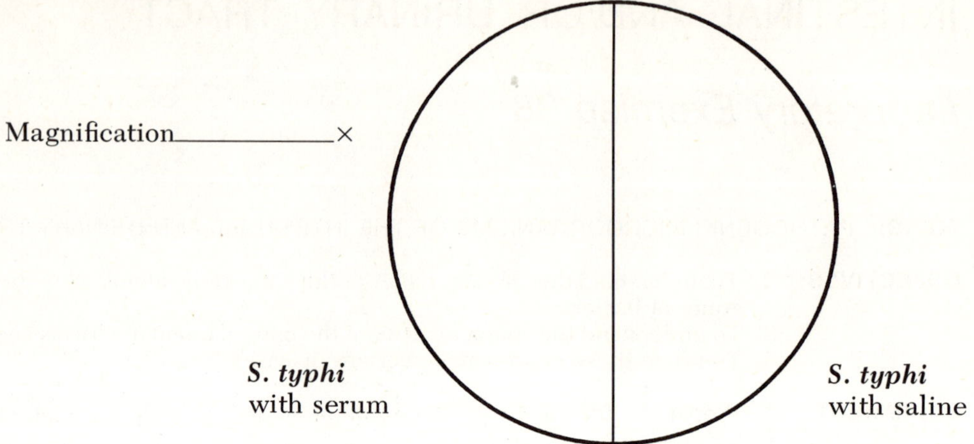

2. Record characteristics of the organisms on the table provided on page 168.

Questions:

1. What is the relationship of *Escherichia coli* to the family *Enterobacteriaceae?*

2. What is the importance of *E. coli?*

3. What are the similarities among the enteric infections?

4. What are the differences among the enteric infections?

5. What are the sanitary factors behind the prevention of enteric infections?

6. What is the importance of poliomyelitis?

   What recent discoveries are significant in the prevention of poliomyelitis?

7. What is the importance of yellow fever?

8. What is the importance of infectious hepatitis?

   How are infectious hepatitis and serum hepatitis related?

   How are these diseases different?

9. What are the public health problems of amebic dysentery?

10. What is the public health significance of undulant fever?

ORGANISMS TRANSMITTED FROM GASTROINTESTINAL AND/OR URINARY TRACT

Organisms*	Specific Morphologic and Cultural Characteristics and Diagnostic Tests	Gram Stain	Disease or Diseases Organism Causes	Methods of Trans-mission	Immu-niza-tion	Specific Precautions to Prevent Transfer
1. GRAM-NEGATIVE RODS Typhoid bacillus *						
Paratyphoid bacillus *						
Dysentery bacillus *						
Colon bacillus *						
2. GRAM-POSITIVE RODS Botulism bacillus *						
Organism of undulant fever *						

*Add the scientific name under the common name of each organism.

ORGANISMS TRANSMITTED FROM GASTROINTESTINAL AND/OR URINARY TRACT

Organisms	Special Characteristics and Diagnostic Tests	Disease Caused	Methods of Transmission	Methods of Prevention	Nursing Responsibilities
3. ENTERIC VIRUSES Virus of polio-myelitis					
Virus of yellow fever					
Virus of infectious hepatitis					
4. ENTERIC PROTOZOA AND METAZOA *Entamoeba histolytica*					
Tapeworm					
Roundworm					
Hookworm					

B. PATHOGENS TRANSMITTED FROM THE RESPIRATORY TRACT

Laboratory Exercise 39

TOPIC: STREPTOCOCCI

OBJECTIVES:
1. To demonstrate the cultural characteristics of certain types of streptococci on blood agar plates.
2. To demonstrate the prevalence of streptococci in the nose and throat.

EQUIPMENT:
1. Sterile defibrinated rabbit or human blood.
2. Sterile 1 ml pipettes.
3. Sterile brain heart infusion agar in tubes for plating.
4. Sterile Petri dishes.
5. Sterile cotton throat swabs.
6. Sterile brain heart infusion broth in tubes.
7. Tongue depressors.
8. Containers of 5 per cent cresol or Lysol.
9. Demonstration of blood agar plates of streptococci showing alpha, beta, and gamma hemolysis.

Procedure:

KEY STEPS	IMPORTANT POINTS
1. Melt the sterile brain heart infusion agar and cool to 45 C.	
2. Obtain a throat culture from your partner.	2.1. Be sure to depress the tongue with a tongue depressor so that you can see the pharynx. 2.2. Have your partner face the light so that you can see the throat clearly. 2.3. Pass a sterile cotton swab through the mouth to the posterior surface of the throat. Avoid the palate and uvula. 2.4. Swab the throat by streaking the cotton-tipped applicator gently over the entire visible surface of the pharynx.
3. Insert the throat swab in a tube of broth.	3.1. Discard the tongue depressor in the cresol or Lysol solution.
4. Wring out the swab on the inside of the tube of brain heart infusion broth.	4.1. Discard the swab in the cresol or Lysol solution.
5. Using a sterile pipette, add 0.5 ml sterile defibrinated blood to the tube of melted, cooled (45 C) sterile brain heart infusion agar. This medium is now called *blood agar.*	5.1. Rotate the heart infusion agar tube to distribute the blood evenly. 5.2. Work rapidly because agar will begin to solidify at 40 C.
6. Transfer a loopful of the culture prepared in Steps 3 and 4 to the tube of blood agar, and pour it into a sterile Petri dish immediately.	6.1. By this technique a poured plate of blood agar will be prepared.

KEY STEPS	**IMPORTANT POINTS**
7. Label the Petri dish and place it in an inverted position in the incubator at 37 C for 24 hr.	7.1. Why place the plate in an inverted position? 7.2. Why should this plate be incubated at 37 C?
8. Remove the plate from the incubator and examine the colonies. Place it in the refrigerator for 24 hr.	8.1. What are the differences in the plate before and after refrigeration.
9. Make smears and Gram stains of several different colonies and examine under the microscope.	
10. Examine demonstration blood agar plates showing alpha, beta and gamma colonies. If these are not readily available, your instructor will show 35 mm projections of blood agar plates.	10.1. Examine with light coming through the plate. 10.2. Examine hemolyzed areas with the low power of the microscope.

Record of Observations:
1. Record descriptions of colonies present on blood agar plates resulting from nose and from throat cultures.
2. Record the results of Gram stains.

Description of Colony	Hemolysis	Gram Stain	Morphologic Types of Organisms

Questions:

1. Define:

   a. Alpha hemolysis

   b. Beta hemolysis

2. What happens to the blood cells in alpha and beta hemolysis? Why?

3. What is the significance of the flora of the nose and throat of individuals without clinical symptoms?

4. When would nose and throat cultures be used for aids in diagnosis?

TOPIC: DEMONSTRATIONS OF MATERIALS ON PATHOGENIC COCCI

1. Observe cultures of *Staphylococcus aureus* and *Staphylococcus epidermidis.*
2. Observe slides showing phagocytized meningococci.

Record of Observations:

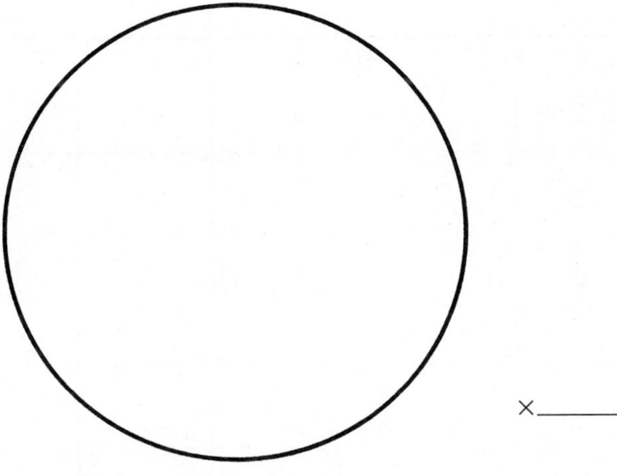

Phagocytized meningococci

Questions:

1. In a suspected case of respiratory infection, why is it important to obtain a specimen of sputum before antibiotic or other specific therapy is started?

2. Why is it especially important to include the source of the specimen when the
meningococcus is the organism suspected of causing the infection?

3. What has happened in phagocytosis?

ORGANISMS TRANSMITTED FROM THE RESPIRATORY TRACT

Organisms*	Specific Morphologic and Cultural Characteristics	Gram Stain	Disease or Diseases the Organism Causes	Methods of Transmission	Immuni-zation	Specific Precautions to Prevent Transfer
1. PATHO-GENIC COCCI Strepto-cocci						
Staphylo-cocci						
Pneumo-cocci						
Meningo-cocci						

*Add the scientific name under the common name of each organism.

LABORATORY IDENTIFICATION OF STAPHYLOCOCCI AND STREPTOCOCCI

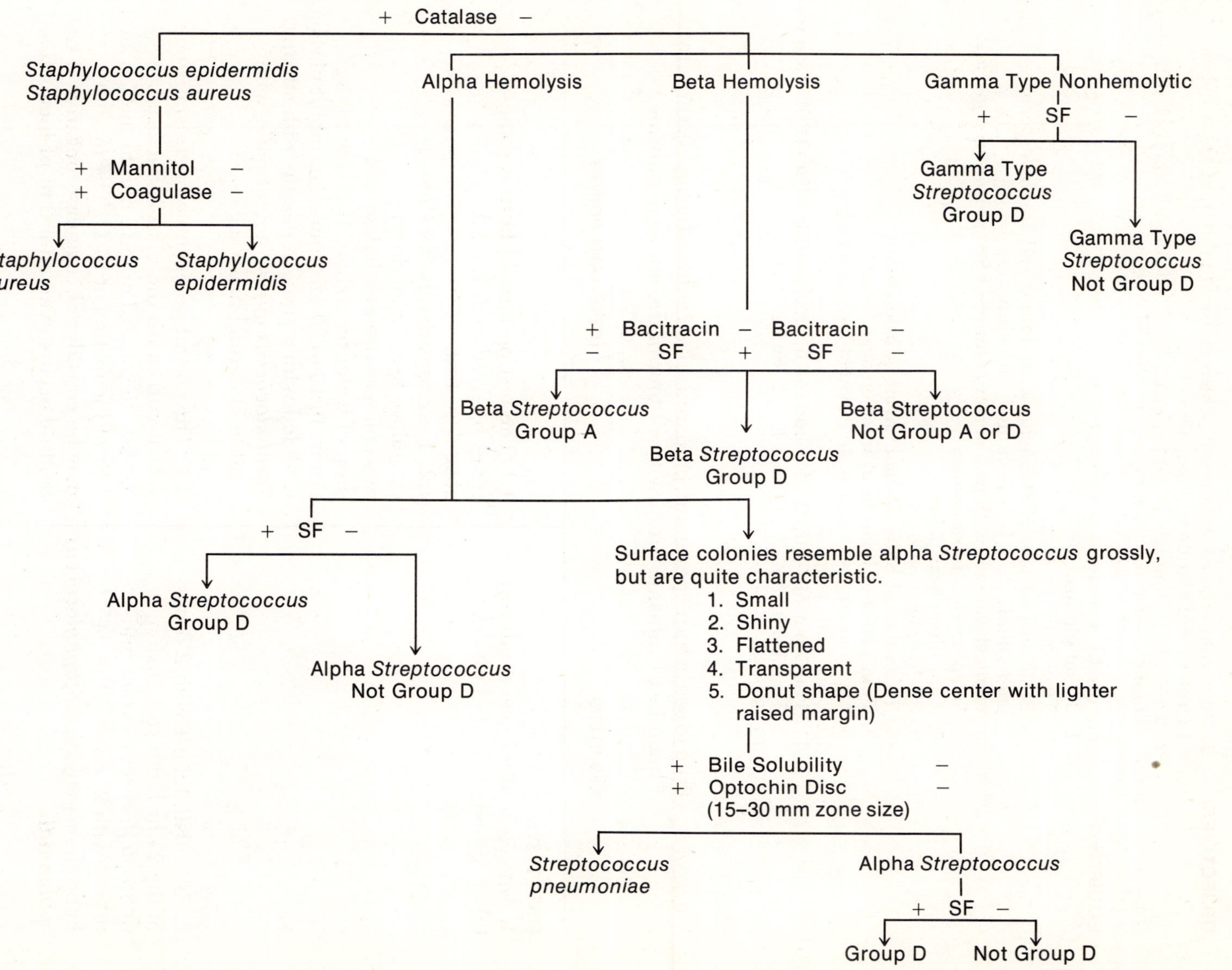

Laboratory Exercise 40

TOPIC: STAPHYLOCOCCI AND STREPTOCOCCI

OBJECTIVES:
1. To perform the coagulase test, which is used to differentiate between virulent and avirulent staphylococci.
2. To study techniques of rapid separations and identification of pathogenic *Staphylococci* and *Streptococci* in clinical specimens.

EQUIPMENT: (For use by 4 students per group)
1. 2.0 ml plasma.
2. Two small test tubes.
3. Broth suspensions of *Staphylococcus aureus* and *Staphylococcus epidermidis* (may be substituted with clinical isolates.)
4. Clinical samples with pus, and/or cultures of *Streptococcus pyogenes*, *Streptococcus pneumoniae*.
5. Four blood agar plates.
6. 3% hydrogen peroxide.
7. Two tubes of buffered brain heart infusion broth.
8. Four plates of brain heart infusion agar.
9. One mannitol salt agar plate (divided into 4 sections).
10. Gram stain reagents.
11. Four optochin (ethylhydrocupreine hydrocholoride) discs (BBL Taxo p).
12. Four bacitracin discs (BBL Taxo A Sensi-disc).
13. Slides.

Procedure: (Prior to use in the experiment, prepare a mixed culture by inoculating a tube of brain heart infusion broth with all four of the above organisms.)

KEY STEPS	IMPORTANT POINTS
FIRST TEST: 1. Into each of the two small test tubes, pipette 0.5 ml of plasma.	1.1 The test performed here is sometimes referred to as the tube coagulase test. 1.2. Less sensitive is the slide coagulase test. To perform it, two colonies are emulsified in a drop of water on a slide. If no clumping occurs in 10 to 20 sec, human or rabbit plasma is added with a straight needle with stirring. *Staphylococcus aureus* agglutinates with visible clumping in 10 sec.
2. Inoculate tube 1 with 2 drops of the 24 hr broth suspension of *Staphylococcus aureus* and tube 2 with 2 drops of the 24 hr broth suspension of *Staphylococcus epidermidis.*	2.1. The coagulase-positive organism is one which will cause the plasma-bacterial mixture to congeal or have clot formation after 1 hr of incubation at 37 C. The mixtures may be considered coagulase-negative if no clotting occurs even after 3 hr of incubation.

KEY STEPSIMPORTANT POINTS

SECOND TEST:

1. From the clinical samples, or the mixture of the four cultures, streak the following plates for isolation and identification.
    a. Four blood agar plates.
    b. Four brain heart infusion agar plates.
    c. One mannitol salt agar plate (divided into four sections).

2. On each of the four blood agar plates put one optochin disc and one bacitracin disc, with a flamed forceps (sterile), over a heavily streaked area of the plate.

2.1. Pneumococci show zones of inhibition 15 to 30 mm in diameter around the optochin discs; other streptococci are not inhibited.

2.2. Bacitracin specifically inhibits group A of the β hemolytic streptococci, but also some α hemolytic streptococci.

3. Incubate the plates for 18 to 24 hr at 37 C.

4. Measure all zones of inhibition of growth (the diameter) in millimeters around the optochin and bacitracin discs. Also note the zones of hemolysis (α, β) or no hemolysis (γ) on the colonies on the blood agar.

4.1. Another test that is specific for only pneumococci is bile solubility. When a few drops of a 10% sodium desoxycholate are added to a growing culture buffered to pH 7.4, lysis of cells occurs within 5 to 10 min. The tube clears completely if the growth is due to the pneumococcus. Other streptococci are not soluble in bile. This test is not part of this exercise, but is mentioned here because it is also valuable in the identification of pneumococci.

5. Observe the growth on the mannitol salt agar.

5.1. Mannitol salt agar is recommended for the selective isolation of pathogenic staphylococci. Why?

5.2. Colonies of pathogenic staphylococci are surrounded by a yellow halo. This shows that mannitol has been fermented.

6. Perform the catalase test on the previously incubated brain heart infusion agar plate by flooding it with 3% hydrogen peroxide.

6.1. The catalase reaction is positive if there is a rapid ebullition of gas.

6.2. Staphylococci and bacilli are catalase positive, streptococci are catalase negative.

7. Make Gram stains from all catalase-positive colonies and all hemolytic (α or β) bacterial colonies.

Record of Observations:

1. Record the results of the coagulase test obtained in the plasma after 1 hr of incubation at 37 C.

COAGULASE TEST

Organism Used	Coagulase Production
Staphylococcus aureus	
Staphylococcus epidermidis	

Questions

1. What laboratory procedure may be used to differentiate between virulent and avirulent staphylococci?

2. What other enzymes or enzyme-like materials are produced by virulent strains of *Staphylococcus aureus*?

3. Why might "false-positive" coagulase tests be reported for certain bacteria or microorganisms that can metabolize citrate?

CULTURAL PROPERTIES OF STAPHYLOCOCCI AND STREPTOCOCCI ON SEVERAL DIFFERENTIAL MEDIA

Medium Used	*Streptococcus pyogenes*	*Streptococcus pneumoniae**	*Staphylococcus aureus*	*Staphylococcus epidermidis*
Blood Agar				
Catalase Test				
Mannitol Salt Agar				
Optochin Disc				
Bacitracin Disc				

*Previously called *Diplococcus pneumoniae.*

Questions:

1. List some of the distinguishing properties of pathogenic strains of **Staphylococcus aureus** which may be observed in the lab experiments just completed.

2. Review possible results for the various differential media used in the experiment and the significance of changes in each type of medium.

3. Explain the importance of being able to rapidly separate and identify pathogenic species of **Staphylococcus** and **Streptococcus** from clinical specimens of patients.

Laboratory Exercise 41

TOPIC: GROWTH OF ANAEROBES

OBJECTIVES: To grow anaerobic organisms in the GasPak anaerobic jar
by the GasPak method.

EQUIPMENT:
1. The GasPak system (a trademark of Becton, Dickinson and Company. It consists of the GasPak 100™ Anaerobic System (vented) which has the following components:
   Polycarbonate anaerobic jar
   Lid (vented)
   O Ring gasket
   Clamp and clamp screw
   Rubber tubing with clamp
   Charged catalyst reaction chamber
   GasPak disposable carbon dioxide generator envelopes
   Disposable anaerobic indicators
2. Blood agar plates and/or thioglycollate medium with glucose and rabbit serum in tubes.
3. Any anaerobic bacteria (from cultures, clinical material, or fresh soil) may be employed as the inoculum. Some facultative anaerobes may be used if strict anaerobes are convenient for the experiment.
4. Palladium-coated alumina pellets.

(A possibility for an experiment is to use three petri plates, one inoculated with a strict anaerobe, one with a facultative organism like **Escherichia coli** or **Staphylococcus aureus,** and one with a strict aerobe such as **Pseudomonas fluorescens.** Strict anaerobes like **Bacteroides fragilis** and some **Clostridium** species are inhabitants of the human intestinal tract.)

Procedure:

KEY STEPS	IMPORTANT POINTS
1. The fresh blood agar plates are streaked with the chosen inoculum with a moist sterile swab.	1.1. Blood agar may consist of trypticase soy agar with 0.5% yeast extract, Vitamin K(menadione)/hemin solution*, and 5% rabbit blood.
2. If desired, cooled (after boiling) thioglycollate medium with glucose and rabbit serum in tubes may be inoculated.	2.1. Other media can be used, such as egg yolk agar for **Clostridium,** or chopped-meat medium for **Bacteroides,** or others.
3. The GasPak disposable hydrogen and carbon dioxide generator envelope eliminates the need for a vacuum pump, gas tanks, etc. It is simple to use and to obtain (BBL, Division of BioQuest, Cockeysville, Maryland 21030).	3.1. Other anaerobic jars may be used for this system, but the GasPak anaerobic jar is most convenient.
4. Palladium-coated alumina pellets (previously heat activated if used before) are placed in screen of the reaction chamber, which is screwed to the inside of the lid.	4.1. The palladium-coated alumina pellets serve as the catalyst for the reaction.

*1 ml per 100 ml medium.

5. The plates and/or tubes are then placed inside the jar. After cutting off the corner of the generator envelope at the dotted line it is placed into the anaerobic jar. The envelope must not be folded or creased.

6. A package containing a disposable anaerobic indicator (methylene blue) is opened, the colored strip is exposed, and the package is placed in the jar so the blue color is visible.

7. 10 ml of tap water are added through the open corner of the envelope with a pipette or syringe. *Never push any object down into the envelope.*

8. Close the anaerobic container (GasPak jar) quickly. Follow special directions if this jar, or another one, is used. It must be airtight.

8.1. The cover (containing the catalyst in a screened reaction chamber in the lid) is placed in position and screwed tight by hand into position.

8.2. Hydrogen is generated in the jar by the following reaction

$$Mg + ZnCl_2 + 2H_2O \xrightarrow{\text{NaOH}} MgCl_2 + Zn(OH)_2 + H_2$$

Then

$$2H_2 + O_2 \xrightarrow{\text{catalyst}} 2H_2O$$

The oxygen is reacting with the hydrogen and the atmosphere becomes anaerobic. This is revealed by the water condensing as a visible mist or fog on the inner wall of the jar. The lid becomes warm. If this does not happen within 25 min, the system is not working properly.

9. After incubation for 3 to 4 hr at 37 C the indicator becomes colorless. Whether incubation time needs to be 24 hr, 48 hr, or longer depends on the organisms that are used.

<table>
<tr><td align="center">KEY STEPS</td><td align="center">IMPORTANT POINTS</td></tr>
<tr><td></td><td>

8.3 *Caution:* Hydrogen gas is explosive.
   a. Have no open flame anywhere near the system.
   b. Check the jars for possible cracks. Do not use faulty jars.
   c. Use a shield around the jar for safety, just in case.
   d. Read directions provided with the jar before you use it.

</td></tr>
</table>

Record of Observations:

Questions:

1. What other systems could you have used to grow bacteria under anaerobic conditions?

Laboratory Exercise 42

TOPIC: BACILLI IN THE RESPIRATORY TRACT

OBJECTIVES: 1. To understand characteristics of pathogenic gram-negative facultatively anaerobic rods and ***Bordetella pertussis*** (now considered to be gram-negative small coccobacilli).
2. To relate these organisms to certain diseases.

EQUIPMENT: 1. Slides of ***Haemophilus influenzae, Bordetella (Haemophilus) pertussis, Yersinia (Pasteurella) pestis,*** or 2 × 2 inch slides of these organisms for projection.*
2. Demonstration of a cough plate from a patient who has whooping cough (***if available.*** This was not difficult so long ago!).

Record of Observations:

1. Observe slides and demonstration plates and fill in the table provided on the next page.

Questions:

1. Is ***H. influenzae*** the causative organism of influenza?

2. What is the community health significance of whooping cough?

---

*It sometimes seems that it is merely to confuse the student, as well as the instructor, that experts keep on changing the names of well recognized pathogens every few years. Note that ***Bordetella pertussis*** and ***Haemophilus pertussis*** are the same organism and ***Yersinia pestis*** is identical to ***Pasteurella pestis.*** Why do you think the classification of bacteria is still being changed?

ORGANISMS TRANSMITTED FROM THE RESPIRATORY TRACT

Organisms*	Specific Morphologic and Cultural Characteristics and Diagnostic Tests	Gram Stain	Disease or Diseases Organism Causes	Methods of Transmission	Immu-niza-tion	Specific Precautions to Prevent Transfer
2. GRAM-NEGATIVE RODS Influenza bacillus						
Whooping cough bacillus						
Organism of bubonic plague						

*Add the scientific name under the common name of each organism.

Laboratory Exercise 43

TOPIC: THE CORYNEBACTERIACEAE AND ACTINOMYCETALES

OBJECTIVES: 1. To understand the characteristics of the pathogenic members of these groups of bacteria.
2. To relate these organisms to certain diseases.

EQUIPMENT: 1. Slides of *Corynebacterium diphtheriae, Mycobacterium tuberculosis, Mycobacterium leprae,* or 35 mm slides for projection.

Record of Observations:

1. Observe slides and fill in the chart provided on the next page.

Questions:

1. How does **C. diphtheriae** enter the body?

2. Where does **C. diphtheriae** grow in a patient who has diphtheria?

3. Why is toxin production important in **C. diphtheriae?**

4. What is the community health significance of tuberculosis?

5. What is the importance of coughing in patients who have tuberculosis?

6. How infectious is Hansen's disease?

ORGANISMS TRANSMITTED FROM THE RESPIRATORY TRACT

Organisms*	Specific Morphologic and Cultural Characteristics and Diagnostic Tests	Special Staining	Disease or Diseases Organism Causes	Methods of Transmission	Immu-niza-tion	Specific Precautions to Prevent Transfer
3. GRAM-POSITIVE RODS Diphtheria bacillus						
3A. ACID-FAST RODS Tubercle bacillus						
Leprosy bacillus						

*Add the scientific name under the common name of each organism.

Laboratory Exercise 44

TOPIC: THE VIRUSES TRANSMITTED FROM THE RESPIRATORY TRACT

OBJECTIVES: 1. To understand the characteristics of pathogenic viruses which are transmitted from the human respiratory tract.
2. To relate these viruses to certain diseases.

EQUIPMENT: 1. Electron micrographs of viruses that affect the respiratory tract.

Record of Observations:

1. Observe the slides and fill in the table provided on the next page.

Questions:

1. What is the community health significance of smallpox?

Why is vaccination against smallpox still important?

Could the smallpox vaccination be dangerous?

2. What is the importance of measles?

Of chickenpox?

3. What are the values of reporting influenza outbreaks?

4. What is the community health significance of encephalitis?

ORGANISMS TRANSMITTED FROM THE RESPIRATORY TRACT

Organisms	Special Characteristics and Diagnostic Tests	Disease Caused	Methods of Transmission	Methods of Prevention	Hospital Responsibilities
4. VIRUSES Virus of smallpox					
Virus of measles					
Virus of influenza					
5. PATHOGENIC* FUNGI Organism of histo-plasmosis					
Organism of coccidioi-domycosis					

*Add the scientific names under the common names of these organisms.

C. PATHOGENS TRANSMITTED FROM THE GENITAL TRACT

Laboratory Exercise 45

TOPIC: THE SPIROCHETES AND GONOCOCCI

OBJECTIVES: 1. To understand the characteristics of the pathogenic members of these groups of organisms.
2. To relate these organisms to certain diseases.

EQUIPMENT: 1. Slides of *Treponema pallidum, Neisseria gonorrhoeae,* or 35 mm slides for projection.

Record of Observations:

1. Observe the slides and fill in the table provided on the next page.

Questions:

1. What is the community health significance of syphilis?

2. How may syphilis be prevented?

3. How may gonorrhea be prevented?

4. Discuss the epidemiology of these diseases at the present time.

PATHOGENS TRANSMITTED FROM THE GENITAL TRACT

Organism	Special Characteristics and Diagnostic Tests	Disease or Diseases the Organism Causes	Methods of Transmission	Immunization	Specific Precautions to Prevent Transfer
1. COCCI Gonococci causes of Vulvovaginitis					
2. Spirochetes *Treponema pallidum*					
3. *Haemophilus ducreyi*					
4. Protozoa *Trichomonas vaginalis*					
5. Viruses (Venereal herpes) (HSV-2)					

D. PATHOGENS FROM THE SOIL

Laboratory Exercise 46

TOPIC: BACTERIA TRANSMITTED FROM THE SOIL

OBJECTIVES: 1. To understand the characteristics of the pathogenic members of the gram-positive bacilli which may be transmitted from the soil.
2. To relate these organisms to certain diseases.

EQUIPMENT: 1. Slides of *Clostridium perfringens, Clostridium tetani, Bacillus anthracis* or 35 mm slides of these organisms for projection.

Record of Observations:

1. Observe the slides and fill in the table provided on the next page.

Questions:

1. How can gas gangrene be prevented?

2. How can tetanus be prevented?

PATHOGENS TRANSMITTED FROM THE SOIL

Organisms*	Specific Morphologic and Cultural Characteristics and Diagnostic Tests	Gram Stain	Disease or Diseases Organism Causes	Methods of Transmission	Immunization	Specific Precautions to Prevent Transfer
1. BACTERIA Gas gangrene bacillus						
Tetanus bacillus						
Anthrax bacillus						

*Add the scientific name under the common name of all organisms.

E. PATHOGENS TRANSMITTED IN THE BLOOD

Laboratory Exercise 47

TOPIC: MICROORGANISMS TRANSMITTED BY BLOOD OR
BY BLOOD-SUCKING INSECTS

OBJECTIVES: 1. To understand the characteristics of the pathogenic members of these groups
of microorganisms.
2. To relate these organisms to certain diseases.

EQUIPMENT: 1. Electron micrograph slides of one of the rickettsias
2. Slides of malarial parasites
3. Slides of *Francisella tularensis (Pasteurella tularensis).*

Record of Observations:

1. Observe the slide and fill in the table provided on the next page.

Questions:

1. In what countries is typhus fever endemic?

   Is this important?
   Why?

2. What is the importance of Rocky Mountain spotted fever?

3. What is the value of insecticides in the control of rickettsial diseases?

4. Why should all dogs be inoculated against rabies?

5. What are the community health problems of malaria?

BLOOD-BORNE PATHOGENS

Organisms	Special Characteristics and Diagnostic Tests	Disease Caused	Methods of Transmission	Methods of Prevention	Hospital Responsibilities
1. BACTERIA Organism of tularemia					
2. RICKETTSIAS *Rickettsia prowazekii*					
Rickettsia rickettsii					
Rickettsia burnetii					
Rickettsia akari					

BLOOD-BORNE PATHOGENS (CONTINUED)

Organisms	Special Characteristics and Diagnostic Tests	Disease Caused	Methods of Transmission	Methods of Prevention	Hospital Responsibilities
3. VIRUSES Virus of homologous serum jaundice					
Virus of encephalitis					
Virus of rabies					
4. PROTOZOA *Plasmodium vivax*					

APPENDIX

GLASSWARE

All glassware used in a laboratory for teaching microbiology should be Kimax or
Pyrex. It is false economy to buy nonheat-resistant glassware for this work because
it is constantly being subjected to high temperatures. Test tubes must be purchased
without lips because lips will collect dust and may be a source of contamination.

Sterile plastic Petri dishes and sterile tubes are available in several sizes
and may be substituted in many experiments where glass Petri dishes or tubes
were used. The plastic labwares are discarded after use, but their cost is relatively
low.

All syringes and needles used must be disposable.

MEDIA

Agar-containing media can be prepared in large flasks. Agar goes into suspension
readily if the distilled water is placed in the flask first and the agar is added to the
water. The flask is then placed in the autoclave and the temperature raised to 121 C.
The steam can be turned off immediately and the pressure in the autoclave reduced
to atmospheric. The agar-containing medium is then in solution and can be tubed
and sterilized. It is always desirable to use flasks with double the volume capacity
of the liquid being sterilized in them.

If flasks are not used for preparing agar medium, it must be prepared in a
double boiler or water bath. Agar will scorch quickly if prepared over direct heat.
Also, if you attempt to prepare nutrient agar in flasks over direct heat, the flasks may
crack and break, resulting in serious burns for anyone who is near the preparation.

Also available in lieu of flasks are "Fleakers." These are hybrids between
flasks and beakers and have the advantages of both. A cover of black rubber-like
plastic fits all "Fleakers" and may be autoclaved separately.

When preparing broth, it is easier to dissolve the dehydrated broth if the
material is added to the water rather than the water to the dehydrated material. If
the broth is heated gently over a direct flame, it can then be tubed and sterilized.

Media can be stored in a refrigerator for six weeks or at room temperature for two
to three weeks.

Information on the composition, preparation, and use of media is available in
printed form from BBL, Colab Laboratories, Difco Laboratories, and Fisher Scientific
Co.

GLASS PETRI DISHES

These can be sterilized in Petri dish cans or can be wrapped in sets of two in
brown paper. *Glass* Petri dishes are best sterilized in the hot air oven. If necessary,
however, the autoclave may be used with a setting of exhaust and dry.

PIPETTES

Pipettes should be loosely stoppered at the mouth end with nonabsorbent cotton. This partially protects the user from accidental contamination of the mouth with cultures or chemicals. Note that special pipettes are being sold that are especially made to hold cotton plugs at the mouth part. Pipettes are most conveniently sterilized in cans in the hot air oven. If necessary they may also be sterilized in the autoclave at a setting of exhaust and dry. The bottom of the can can be lined with a layer of glass wool to protect the tips of the pipettes. If pipette cans are not available, pipettes can be wrapped singly or in pairs in brown wrapping paper and sterilized in the hot air oven. Disposable sterile pipettes may also be purchased, wrapped in plastic. They are not too expensive for small scale laboratory work.

Pathogens should not be pipetted by mouth. Bulbs of different makes and types are available that can be used with only one hand after they are attached to the top of the pipette. All of these devices are quite simple to use and make pipetting perfectly safe. See your local supplier about them.

POURING LARGE NUMBERS OF PLATES

It is sometimes more convenient for instructors and students to have large numbers of plates poured before certain laboratory periods. Agar medium can be prepared in 1,000 ml amounts in large flasks. After sterilizing these flasks of agar in the autoclave for 15 min, they can be removed from the autoclave and cooled to approximately 50 C. Sterile Petri dishes can be placed on a laboratory desk in stacks of four. After removing the cotton stopper from the flask, flame the mouth of the flask, grasp four Petri dishes in the left hand, raise the cover of the bottom dish and pour in enough agar medium to cover the bottom of the dish. Lower the cover of this Petri dish and raise the cover of the next Petri dish in the stack. Continue in this way until all the Petri dishes are poured. Flame the mouth of the flask after pouring every four Petri dishes. Leave the Petri dishes in stacks of four until the agar has hardened.

STAINS

Stains used in microbiology should be made up fresh every four to six weeks. They may be dispensed in staining bottles containing droppers with a bulb.

STORAGE IN INCUBATOR OR REFRIGERATOR

If small test tubes (10 × 77 mm) are used for cultures, they can be placed in small fruit juice or soup cans for incubation. The bottoms of the cans should be lined with cotton to prevent fracture of the tubes. The use of these cans conserves space in the incubator and/or refrigerator.

ROUTINE STUDY OF PURE CULTURES

After an organism has been isolated into pure culture it becomes necessary to determine various characteristics in order to distinguish it from other more or less closely related forms.

The basic features that need to be observed include:

I. Morphology

1. Microscopic
   a. shape, size, cell grouping
   b. presence or absence of spores
   c. motility, arrangement of flagella on motile forms
   d. capsules
   e. staining reactions—Gram's stain and special stains

2. Cultural
   a. appearance of colonies (size, shape, color, and so on)
   b. appearance of broth cultures
   c. appearance on special media

II. Biochemical and Physiological Reactions

1. Fermentation of carbohydrates, alcohols, glucosides, and so on

2. Proteolytic activity as measured by the effect on gelatin

3. Formation of indol

4. Nitrate reduction

5. Production of hydrogen sulfide

6. Special tests—Voges-Proskauer reaction, hemolysis of blood, action on milk, and so on

7. Relation to free oxygen

8. Temperature relations

The information developed by these observations supplies a great deal of knowledge about any given culture. For complete classification additional tests may be required, and in some instances pathogenic properties or immunologic reactions are of service in differentiating closely related species.

In order to facilitate the study of significant characteristics in a systematic way the American Society for Microbiology through its Committee on Bacteriological Technic sponsors a ***Manual of Microbiologic Methods,**** and makes available a standard descriptive chart. Descriptions of the known bacterial species and keys for identification are available in ***Bergey's Manual of Determinative Bacteriology.***†

The following outline, based in part upon the simplified descriptive chart of the American Society for Microbiology, includes the salient features of pure culture study and the descriptive terminology that should be used.

---

*Society of American Bacteriologists, Committee on Bacteriological Technic: Manual of Microbiologic Methods. 1957, New York, McGraw-Hill Book Co., Inc.
†Bergey's Manual of Determinative Bacteriology, 8th Ed. 1974, Baltimore, The Williams & Wilkins Co.

Name of organism ____

Source_____________________ Habitat_____________________________

Medium___________________ Age _________________________________

CELL MORPHOLOGY: cocci, rods, vibrios, spirals, branched rods or filaments

VEGETATIVE CELLS: form and arrangement

      Cocci—spherical cells
      Streptococci—cells in chains
      Diplococci—cells in pairs
      Micrococci—cells singly
      Sarcinae—cells in cubes
      Staphylococci—cells in irregular clusters
      Tetrads—cells in fours
      Rods—cylindrical cells
      Coccobacilli—flattened spherical cells

      Include cell arrangement, size (long rods, short rods, etc.)
      Ends:

SPORANGIA: cells containing spores. Age _______________________________

    None, or if present note shape:
      Rods—not different from vegetative cell
        Rounded—an arc of a circle
        Truncate—square
        Concave—hollow and curved
        Tapering—spindle shaped
      Spindles—larger in middle than at ends
      Elliptical—in form of an ellipse
      Clavate—club shaped
      Drumstick—one end enlarged

ENDOSPORES:

      Shape—spherical, ellipsoidal or cylindrical
      Position—central to eccentric, terminal or subterminal

Irregular or Pleomorphic Forms:

      Record medium and age of culture

Motility in broth _______________________ Arrangement of flagella _____________

Staining Characteristics:

Gram __________________________ Age _________________________________

      Special stains, as volutin, fat, acid fast, capsule

CULTURAL FEATURES:

Agar Slant   Age _______________________

    Amount of growth—scanty, moderate, or abundant

    Form:
        filiform—uniform along line of inoculation
        echinulate—toothed or pointed margins
        beaded—separate or confluent colonies along line of inoculation
        spreading—growth extending several millimeters beyond line of inoculation
        rhizoid—irregular, branched or rootlike in character
        arborescent—branched, treelike growth

    Consistency:
        butyrous—butter-like
        viscid—growth follows needle when withdrawn
        membranous—thin, coherent, like a membrane
        brittle—dry, friable

    Chromogenesis: none, or if present indicate color

    Optical Characters:
        opaque—not permitting light to pass through
        translucent—some light passes through but not enough to permit visibility of
                objects viewed through growth
        opalescent—like an opal in color
        iridescent—exhibiting changing rainbow colors in reflected light
        fluorescent—having one color by reflected light and another by transmitted
                 light
        dull—not glossy
        glistening—glossy

    Odor: absent, or resembling _________________________________

    Medium Change: record color change in medium if present

Agar Colonies   Age ___________________

    Form:
        punctiform—under 1 mm in diameter
        circular
        filamentous—long, irregular placed or interwoven threads
        rhizoid—irregular branched or rootlike in character
        irregular

    Elevation:
        effuse—thin, veily, unusually spreading
        flat
        raised—thick, with abrupt or terraced edges
        convex—segment of a circle but flattened

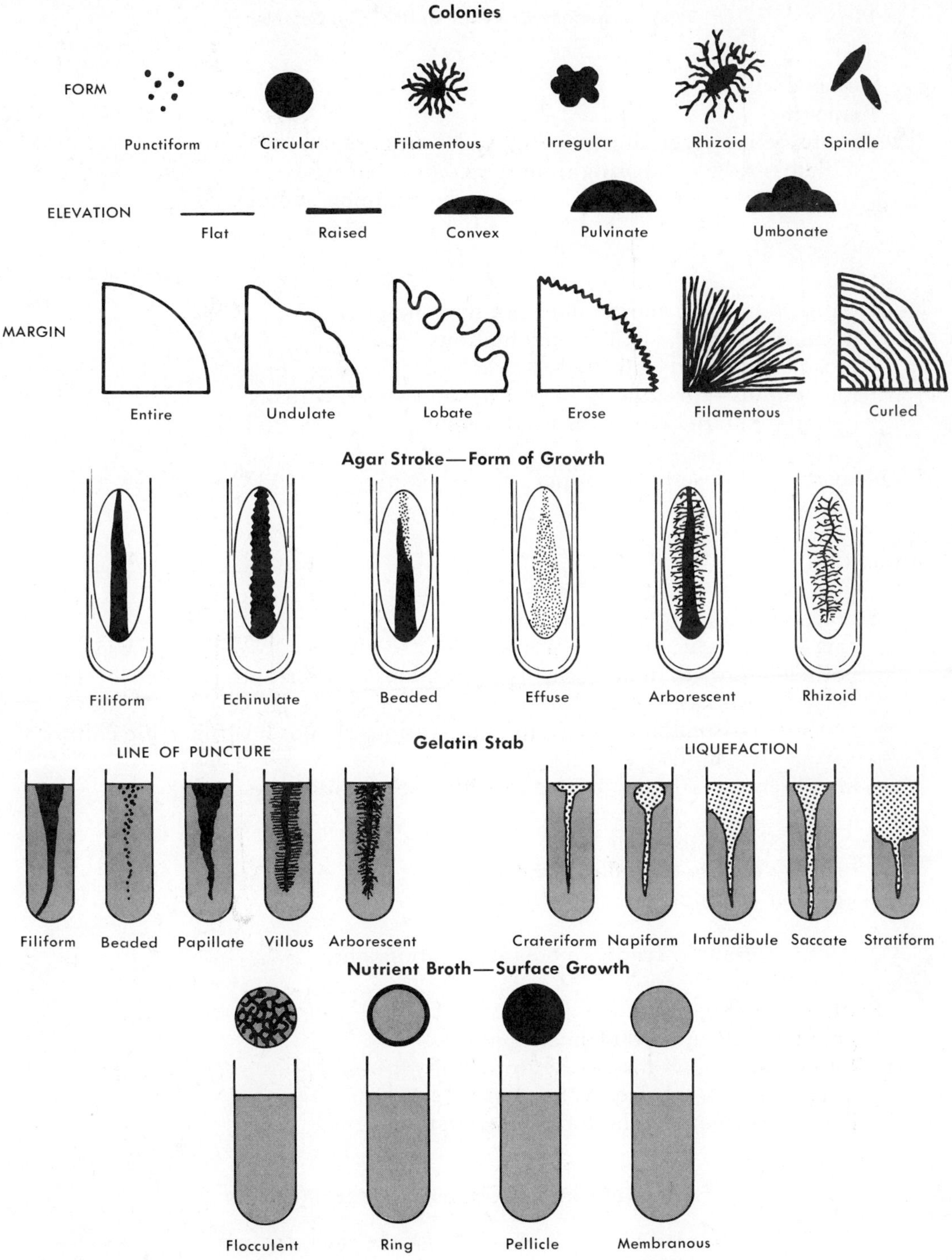

Colonies

FORM

Punctiform   Circular   Filamentous   Irregular   Rhizoid   Spindle

ELEVATION

Flat   Raised   Convex   Pulvinate   Umbonate

MARGIN

Entire   Undulate   Lobate   Erose   Filamentous   Curled

Agar Stroke—Form of Growth

Filiform   Echinulate   Beaded   Effuse   Arborescent   Rhizoid

Gelatin Stab

LINE OF PUNCTURE

Filiform   Beaded   Papillate   Villous   Arborescent

LIQUEFACTION

Crateriform   Napiform   Infundibule   Saccate   Stratiform

Nutrient Broth—Surface Growth

Flocculent   Ring   Pellicle   Membranous

*From *Manual of Microbiological Methods,* Committee on Microbiological Technique, Society of American Bacteriologists, McGraw-Hill Book Co., New York.

Types of Surface Elevation of Bacterial Colonies

Surface:
  smooth
  contoured—irregular, smoothly undulating, like a relief map
  radiate—ridges radiating from the center like spokes in a wheel
  concentric—marked with rings having common center
  rugose—wrinkled

Margin:
  entire—smooth, margin does not have notches
  undulate—wavy, shallow indentations
  erose—irregularly notched
  filamentous—irregularly placed or interwoven threads
  curled—parallel chains in wavy strands

Density: See description of optical characters

Nutrient Broth   Age _____________________

  Surface growth: none, or
    ring—growth at upper margin adherent to glass
    pellicle—growth in the form of a continuous or interrupted sheet over the
        surface
    flocculent—small masses of growth of various shapes floating in the culture
        fluid
    membranous—thin, coherent growth like a membrane

  Subsurface growth: none, or
    turbid—cloudy with flocculent particles
    granular—composed of small granules

  Amount of growth: scanty, moderate or abundant

  Sediment: none, or
    granular—composed of small granules
    flocculent—small masses of growth of various shapes
    viscid—sediment rises as a coherent swirl
    flaky—sediment in the form of separate flakes

Types of Surface Elevation of Bacterial Colonies

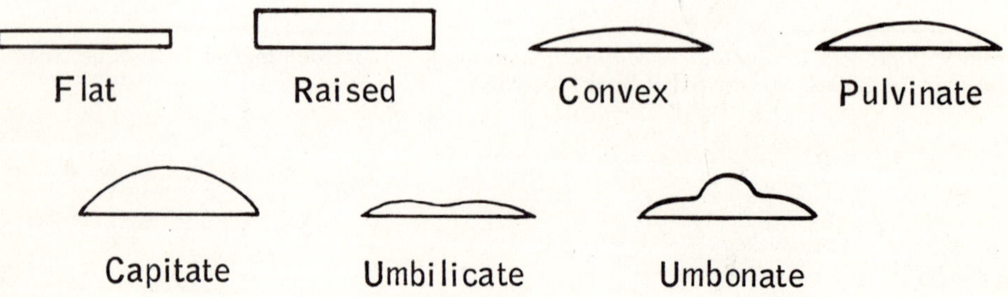

Gelatin Stab   Age _______________________

 Liquefaction or none
 Note: The shape of the area of liquefaction in gelatin cultures incubated at 25 C
         may have significance
 Rate: slow, moderate, or rapid

Milk   Indicator _______________________

 Indicate the change observed and the day on which it became apparent

 Include:
    reaction—unchanged, acid, alkaline
    curd—acid or rennent
    peptonization—digestion of casein
    reduction of indicator

Fermentation of Carbohydrates

 Indicate medium, whether acid and, if acid, whether gas is also formed

Action on Nitrates   Medium _______________________

 Nitrate—day on which positive
 Gas (N)—day on which positive

Hydrogen Sulfide Production   Medium _______________________

 Record as positive or negative

Indole Production   Medium _______________________

 Age _______________________

 Method _______________________

 Record as positive or negative

Relation to Free Oxygen

 Medium _______________ Age _______________________________________

 Method _______________

 Aerobic growth: Absent, present, better than anaerobic growth, poorer than
    anaerobic growth

 Anaerobic growth: present or absent

Temperature Relations

Record temperatures tested and whether growth is present or lacking

Special Tests

Record medium, nature and result of test or observation for such features as Methyl red test, Voges-Proskauer reaction, Triple Sugar Iron Agar, Endo's medium, Lewis-Pittman medium, blood agar, starch agar, or such others as may be required. An explanation of the medium to be used and the test to be done will be given by the laboratory instructor when necessary.

After the results of the various tests and observations have been recorded it is advisable to check against the description given in *Bergey's Manual.* More detailed study of the unknown species may be required before positive identification can be made by tracing the organism through the taxonomic keys given in *Bergey's Manual.*

Student_______________________________________

Lab Section____________________________________

Date Started___________________________________

Date Completed_________________________________

Routine Study of Pure Cultures

MORPHOLOGICAL CHARACTERISTICS		DESCRIPTIVE CHART				
Cell Shape:		Organism:_________________________				
Arrangement:		PHYSIOLOGICAL CHARACTERISTICS				
Size:						
Spores:		TESTS		RESULTS		
Gram Stain:						
Motility:		Fermentation:		24 hr	48 hr	72 hr
Capsules:		Glucose				
Special Stains:		Lactose				
		Sucrose				
CULTURAL CHARACTERISTICS		Gelatin Liquefaction				
Colonies:		Litmus Milk	Acid / Alk / Coag / red'n / Pept			
form						
elevation						
surface		Reaction:				
margin		Age:				
Agar Slant:		Indole				
amount of growth						
form		Nitrate Reduction				
consistency		Hydrogen Sulfide				
optical characteristics						
Nutrient Broth:		Starch Hydrolysis				
surface		Citrate Utilization				
substance						
amount		Acetylmethyl Carbinol				
sediment		Methyl Red Test				
Blood Agar:		Urease				
Gelatin Stab:						
Oxygen Requirements:						
Optimum Temperature:						

(Additional copies of this form appear on pages 211–214.)

DIFFERENTIATION OF ENTEROBACTERIACEAE BY BIOCHEMICAL TESTS†

	Escherichieae		Edwardsielleae	Salmonelleae				Klebsielleae								Proteeae					
TEST or SUBSTRATE	Escherichia	Shigella	Edwardsiella	Salmonella	Arizona	Citrobacter	Klebsiella	Enterobacter						Serratia	Pectobacterium	Proteus				Providencia	
								cloacae	aerogenes	hafniae 37C	hafniae 22C	liquefaciens 37C	liquefaciens 22C		25C	vulgaris	mirabilis	morganii	rettgeri	alcalifaciens	stuartii
Indol	+	−or+	+	−	−	−	−or+	−	−	−	−	−	−	−	−or+	+	−	+	+	+	+
Methyl Red	+	+	+	+	+	+	−	−	−	+or−	−	+or−	−or+	−or+	+or−	+	+	+	+	+	+
Voges-Proskauer	−	−	−	−	−	−	+	+	+	+or−	+	−or+	+or−	+	−or+	−	−or+	−	−	−	−
Simmons' Citrate	−	−	−	d	+	+	+	+	+	(+)or−	d	+	+	+	d	d	+or(+)	−	+	+	+
Hydrogen Sulfide (TSI)	−	−	+	+	+	+or−	−	−	−	−	−	−	−	−	−	+	+	−	−	−	−
Urease	−	−	−	−	−	d w	+	+or−	−	−	−	d	−	d w	d w	+	+	+	+	−	−
KCN	−	−	−	−	−	+	+	+	+	+	+	+	+	+	+or−	+	+	+	+	+	+
Motility	+or−	−	+	+	+	+	−	+	+	+	+	d	+	+	+or−	+	+	+	+	+	+
Gelatin (22C)	−	−	−	−	(+)	−	−	(+)or−	−or(+)		−		+	+	+or(+)	+or(+)	+	−	−	−	−
Lysine Decarboxylase	d	−	+	+	+	−	+	−	+	+	+	+or−	+	+	−	−	−	−	−	−	−
Arginine Dihydrolase	d	−or(+)	−	(+)or+	+or(+)	d	−	+	−	−	−	−	−	−	−or+	−	−	−	−	−	−
Ornithine Decarboxylase	d	d[1]	+	+	+	d	−	+	+	+	+	+	+	+	−	−	+	+	−	−	+
Phenylalanine Deaminase	−	−	−	−	−	−	−	−	−	−	−	−	−	−	−	+	+	+	+	+	+
Malonate	−	−	−	−	+	d	+	+or−	+or−	+or−	+or−	−	−	−	−or+	−or+	−	−	−	−	−
Gas from Glucose	+	−[1]	+	+	+	+	+	+	+	+	+	+	+	+or−[3]	−or+	+or−	+	d	−or+	+or−	−
Lactose	+	−[1]	−	−	d	d	+	+	+	−or(+)	−or(+)	d	(+)	−or(+)	d	−	−	−	−	−	−
Sucrose	d	−[1]	−	−	−	d	+	+	+	d	d	+	+	+	+	+	+	d	−	d	d
Mannitol	+	+or−	−	+	+	+	+	+	+	+	+	+	+	+	+	+	−	−	+or−	−	d
Dulcitol	d	d	−	d[2]	−	d	−or+	−or+	−	−	−	−	−	−	−	−	−	−	d	−	−
Salicin	d	−	−	−	−	d	+	+or(+)	+	d	d	+	+	+	+	d	d	−	d	−	−
Adonitol	−	−	−	−	−	−	+or−	−or+	+	−	−	d	d	d	−	−	−	−	d	+	−
Inositol	−	−	−	d	−	−	+	d	+	−	−	+	+	d	−	−	−	−	+	−	+
Sorbitol	+	d	−	+	+	+	+	+	+	−	−	+	+	+	−	−	−	−	d	−	d
Arabinose	+	d	−	+[2]	+	+	+	+	+	+	+	+	+	−	+	−	−	−	−	−	−
Raffinose	d	d	−	−	−	d	+	+	+	−	−	+	+	−	+or(+)	−	−	−	−	−	−
Rhamnose	d	d	−	+	+	+	+	+	+	+	+	−	−	−	d	−	−	−	+or−	−	−

[1] Formerly *Escherichia freundii*.
[2] *S. typhi, S. pullorum, S. paratyphi-A, S. choleraesuis,* and a few others do not ferment dulcitol promptly, *S. choleraesuis* does not ferment arabinose
+ Positive 1 or 2 days   X Late and irregularly positive   − Negative   d Different biochemical types
(+) Delayed positive reaction
* Certain biotypes of *S. flexneri* 6 produce gas; *S. sonnei* cultures ferment lactose and sucrose slowly and decarboxylate ornithine

(From BBL, Division of Becton, Dickinson and Company. After Ewing: Biochemical Reactions Given by the Enterobacteriaceae in Commonly Used Tests. Enteric Bacteriology Laboratories, DHEW-HSMHA-NCDC, Atlanta, Ga. 30333. October 1969. Reprinted by permission.)
†For another system of differentiation see the next page.

THE ENTEROTUBE SYSTEM

Another system for the differentiation of Enterobacteriaceae by biochemical tests is the Enterotube, a prepared, sterile multimedia tube for the rapid differential identification of gram-negative bacteria, manufactured by Hoffmann-La Roche, Inc., and available from your local supplier. Instructions for performing the test come with each shipment.

A table showing reactions of various gram-negative bacteria with the Enterotube is shown below.

Group	Genus	Species	Dextrose (Glucose)	Gas Production from Glucose	Lysine Decarboxylase	Ornithine Decarboxylase	H$_2$S	Indole	Lactose	Dulcitol	Phenylalanine Deaminase	Urea	Simmons Citrate
Escherichieae	Escherichia		+ 100.0	+K 92.0	d 80.6	d 57.8	−L 0.0	+ 96.3	+K 91.6	d 49.3	− 0.0	− 0.0	− 0.2
Escherichieae	Shigella		+ 100.0	−A 2.1	− 0.0	∓B 20.0	− 0.0	∓ 39.8	−B 0.3	d 5.4	− 0.0	− 0.0	− 0.0
Edwardsielleae	Edwardsiella		+ 100.0	+ 99.4	+ 100.0	+ 99.7	+ 99.7	+ 99.1	− 0.0	− 0.0	− 0.0	− 0.0	− 0.0
Salmonelleae	Salmonella		+ 100.0	+C 91.9	+H 94.6	+I 92.7	+E 91.6	− 1.1	− 0.8	dD 86.5	− 0.0	− 0.0	dF 80.1
Salmonelleae	Arizona		+ 100.0	+ 99.3	+ 100.0	+ 100.0	+ 99.0	− 3.5	d 66.3	− 0.0	− 0.0	− 0.0	+ 98.7
Salmonelleae	Citrobacter	freundii	+ 100.0	+ 90.9	− 0.0	d 30.7	± 81.6	∓ 21.9	d 38.3	d 58.7	− 0.0	dw 70.8	+ 90.4
Salmonelleae	Citrobacter	diversus	+ 100.0	+ 97.3	− 0.0	+ 100.0	− 0.0	+ 100.0	d 32.7	± 53.1	− 0.0	dw 77.9	+ 99.1
Proteeae	Proteus	vulgaris	+ 100.0	±G 86.0	− 0.0	− 0.0	+ 94.7	+ 91.4	− 0.0	− 0.0	+ 100.0	+ 94.7	d 10.5
Proteeae	Proteus	mirabilis	+ 100.0	+G 93.4	− 0.0	+ 98.4	+ 94.2	− 3.2	− 1.5	− 0.0	+ 99.6	+ 88.4	+ 58.7
Proteeae	Proteus	morganii	+ 100.0	±G 84.9	− 0.0	+ 95.7	− 0.0	+ 99.5	− 0.0	− 0.0	+ 95.0	+ 97.1	−J 0.0
Proteeae	Proteus	rettgeri	+ 100.0	∓G 12.2	− 0.0	− 0.0	− 0.0	+ 95.9	d 10.0	− 0.0	+ 98.0	+ 100.0	+ 95.6
Proteeae	Providencia	alcalifaciens	+ 100.0	dG 85.2	− 0.0	− 1.2	− 0.0	+ 99.4	− 0.3	− 0.0	+ 97.4	− 0.0	+ 97.9
Proteeae	Providencia	stuartii	+ 100.0	− 0.0	− 0.0	− 0.0	− 0.0	+ 98.6	− 3.6	− 0.0	+ 94.5	− 0.0	+ 95.6
Klebsielleae	Enterobacter	cloacae	+ 100.0	+ 99.3	− 0.0	+ 93.7	− 0.0	− 0.0	+ 76.3	d 15.2	− 0.0	± 74.6	+ 98.9
Klebsielleae	Enterobacter	aerogenes	+ 100.0	+ 95.9	+ 97.5	+ 95.9	− 0.0	− 0.8	+ 92.5	− 4.1	− 0.0	− 5.0	+ 92.6
Klebsielleae	Enterobacter	hafniae	+ 100.0	+ 98.9	+ 99.6	+ 98.6	− 0.0	− 0.0	d 2.8	− 2.4	− 0.0	− 6.6	d 5.6
Klebsielleae	Enterobacter agglomerans	aerogenic	+ 100.0	+ 100.0	− 0.0	− 0.0	− 0.0	∓ 37.2	+ 85.0	d 52.2	∓ 15.9	d 40.0	d 61.9
Klebsielleae	Enterobacter agglomerans	anaerogenic	+ 100.0	− 0.0	− 0.0	− 0.0	− 0.0	∓ 13.7	d 28.6	− 1.4	∓ 31.1	d 24.8	+ 67.8
Klebsielleae	Serratia	marcescens	+ 100.0	±G 52.6	+ 99.6	+ 99.6	− 0.0	−w 0.2	− 1.3	− 0.0	− 0.0	dw 39.7	+ 97.6
Klebsielleae	Serratia	liquefaciens	+ 100.0	d 72.5	+ 64.2	+ 100.0	− 0.0	−w 1.8	d 15.6	− 0.0	− 0.9	dw 3.7	+ 93.6
Klebsielleae	Serratia	rubidaea	+ 100.0	dG 35.0	+ 61.0	− 0.0	− 0.0	−w 2.0	+ 100.0	− 0.0	− 0.0	dw 4.0	+ 88.0
Klebsielleae	Klebsiella	pneumoniae	+ 100.0	+ 96.0	+ 97.2	− 0.0	− 0.0	− 6.8	+ 98.7	∓ 33.0	− 0.0	+ 95.4	+ 96.8
Klebsielleae	Klebsiella	ozaenae	+ 100.0	d 55.0	∓ 35.8	− 4.0	− 0.0	− 0.0	d 26.2	− 0.0	− 0.0	d 14.8	d 28.1
Klebsielleae	Klebsiella	rhinoschleromatis	+ 100.0	− 0.0	− 0.0	− 0.0	− 0.0	− 0.0	d 6.0	− 0.0	− 0.0	− 0.0	− 0.0
Yersineae		enterocolitica	+ 100.0	− 0	− 0	+ 90.7	− 0	∓ 26.7	− 0	− 0	− 0	+ 90.7	− 0
Yersineae		pseudotuberculosis	+ 100.0	− 0	− 0	− 0	− 0	− 0	− 0	− 0	− 0	+ 100	− 0

Percentage Chart—Reaction Legend

Numbers indicate percentage of strains giving positive reactions within 24-hour incubation.

+ Positive   − Negative   ± Majority Positive   ∓ Majority Negative   d Different Biochemical Types

w Weak Reaction

A. Certain biotypes of *S. flexneri* 6 form gas.
B. *S. sonnei* strains usually ferment lactose slowly (3 days or longer) and are not likely to be positive in ENTEROTUBE. Cultures of this species decarboxylate ornithine.
C. *S. typhi* and *S. gallinarum* are anaerogenic.
D. *S. typhi, S. cholerae-suis, S. enteritidis* bioserotypes Paratyphi A and Pullorum, and a few others do not ferment dulcitol promptly.
E. *S. enteritidis* bioserotype Paratyphi A and some rare biotypes may be H$_2$S-negative.
F. *S. typhi, S. enteritidis* bioserotype Paratyphi A and some rare biotypes are citrate-negative and *S. cholerae-suis* is usually delayed positive.
G. The amount of gas produced by *Serratia, Proteus* and *Providencia alcalifaciens* is slight; therefore, gas production may not be evident in the ENTEROTUBE.
H. *S. enteritidis* bioserotype Paratyphi A is negative for lysine decarboxylase.
I. *S. typhi* and *S. gallinarum* are ornithine decarboxylase-negative.
J. Use ornithine, H$_2$S and indole for speciation of *P. morganii* since false-positive citrate reactions may occur occasionally.
K. The Alkalescens-Dispar (A-D) group are included as biotypes of *E. coli.* Members of the A-D group are generally anaerogenic, nonmotile and do not ferment lactose.
L. An occasional strain may produce hydrogen sulfide.

SOURCE OF MATERIALS AND EQUIPMENT

CULTURES

1. Local hospital or Pathology laboratory

2. American Type Culture Collection
   12301 Parklawn Drive
   Rockville, Md. 20852

SLIDES (PREPARED FOR MICROSCOPIC STUDY AND/OR PROJECTION)

1. Ward's Natural Science
   Establishment, Inc.
   P.O. Box 1712
   Rochester, N.Y. 14603

   P.O. Box 1749
   Monterey, Calif. 93940

2. American Society for Microbiology
   Dr. Helen L. Bishop
   1913 I St., N.W.
   Washington, D.C. 20006

For Biochrome Mounts (35 mm color slides)

3. Elliot Scientific Corp.
   185 East 85th Street
   New York, N.Y. 10028

MEDIA

1. Difco Laboratories
   P.O. Box 1058A
   Detroit, Mich. 48232

2. Preweighed bacteriological media
   available from
   Fisher Laboratories
   585 Alpha Dr.
   Pittsburgh, Pa. 15238

3. BBL—Division of BioQuest
   P.O. Box 243
   Cockeysville, Md. 21030

LABORATORY EQUIPMENT

1. Ward's Natural Science Establishment, Inc.
   P.O. Box 1712
   Rochester, N.Y. 14603

P.O. Box 1749
Monterey, Calif. 93940

2. VWR Scientific/Treck Photographic
   7230 Mykawa Road
   P.O. Box 33348
   Houston, Tex. 77033

3. Fisher Scientific Co.
   1600 W. Glenlake Ave.
   P.O. Box 171
   Itasca, Ill. 60143

   5481 Creek Rd.
   Cincinnati, Ohio 45242

   461 Riverside Ave.
   Medford, Mass. 02155

   1241 Ambassador Blvd.
   St. Louis, Mo. 63132

   8505 Devonshire Rd.
   Montreal 307, Quebec, Canada

   Also in:
   Washington, D.C.
   Raleigh
   Atlanta
   Cleveland
   Rochester
   New York
   Houston
   Philadelphia
   Mexico
   Puerto Rico
   Ottawa
   Toronto
   Vancouver
   Zurich
   Others

4. Central Scientific Co.
   Div. of Cenco Instruments Corp.
   2600 South Kostner Ave.
   Chicago, Ill. 60623

5. Arthur H. Thomas Co.
   P.O. Box 779
   Vine Street at Third
   Philadelphia, Pa. 19105

6. Curtin Matheson Scientific Inc.
   4220 Jefferson Avenue
   P.O. Box 1546
   Houston, Tex. 77001

   10727 Tucker Street
   Beltsville, Md. 20705

   For Chicago:
   1850 Greenleaf Ave.
   Elk Grove Village, Ill. 60007

   For San Francisco:
   470 Valley Drive
   P.O. Box 386
   Brisbane, Calif. 94005

   7524 Currency Drive
   P.O. Box 13930
   Orlando Central Park
   Orlando, Florida 32809

   Also in:
   Atlanta
   Boston
   Dallas
   Los Angeles
   Midland, Mich.
   Minneapolis
   New Orleans
   St. Louis
   Tulsa
   Wayne, N.J.
   Washington, D.C.
   Monterrey, Mexico
   Cincinnati
   Others

7. Mallinckrodt Chemical Works
   2nd & Mallinckrodt Streets
   P.O. Box 5439
   St. Louis, Mo. 63160

8. Bellco Biological Glassware
   340 Edrudo Road
   Vineland, N.J. 08360

9. Scientific Products
   For Dallas:
   210 Great Southwest Parkway
   Grand Prairie, Tex. 75050

1210 Waukegan Road
McGaw Park, Ill. 60085

8855 McGaw Road
Columbia, Md. 21045

For Los Angeles:
   P.O. Box C19505
   17111 Red Hill Avenue
   Irvine, Calif. 92705

Also in:
   Columbus
   New Orleans
   Edison, N.J.
   St. Louis
   San Francisco
   Seattle
   Minneapolis
   Miami
   Houston
   North Kansas City, Mo.
   Charlotte, N.C.
   Detroit
   Boston
   Atlanta
   Others

10. Sargent-Welch Scientific Co.
    35 Stern Avenue
    Springfield, N.J. 07081

    5915 Peeler Street
    Dallas, Tex. 75235

    P.O. Box 7196
    Denver, Colo. 80207

    8560 West Chicago Avenue
    Detroit, Mich. 48204

    9520 Midwest Avenue
    Garfield Heights
    Cleveland, Ohio 44125

    10400 Taconic Terrace
    Cincinnati, Ohio 45215

    P.O. Box 10404
    Birmingham, Ala. 35202

1617 East Ball Road
Anaheim, Calif. 92803

7300 North Linder Avenue
Skokie, Ill. 60076

285 Garyray Drive, Weston
Toronto, Ontario, Canada

3300 Cavendish Blvd.
Montreal, Quebec, Canada

11. Millipore Intertech Inc.
P.O. Box 255
Bedford, Mass. 01730

12. Carolina Biological Supply Co.
2700 York Road
Burlington, N.C. 27215

13. Grand Island Biological Company
3175 Staley Road
Grand Island, N.Y. 14072

519 Aldo Avenue
Santa Clara, Calif. 95050

Student_______________________________________

Lab Section___________________________________

Date Started__________________________________

Date Completed_______________________________

Routine Study of Pure Cultures

MORPHOLOGICAL CHARACTERISTICS		DESCRIPTIVE CHART					
Cell Shape:		Organism:_________________________					
Arrangement:		PHYSIOLOGICAL CHARACTERISTICS					
Size:							
Spores:		TESTS		RESULTS			
Gram Stain:							
Motility:		Fermentation:		24 hr	48 hr	72 hr	
Capsules:		Glucose					
Special Stains:		Lactose					
		Sucrose					
CULTURAL CHARACTERISTICS		Gelatin Liquefaction					
Colonies:		Litmus Milk	Acid	Alk	Coag	red'n	Pept
form							
elevation							
surface		Reaction:					
margin		Age:					
Agar Slant:		Indole					
amount of growth							
form		Nitrate Reduction					
consistency		Hydrogen Sulfide					
optical characteristics							
Nutrient Broth:		Starch Hydrolysis					
surface		Citrate Utilization					
substance		Acetylmethyl Carbinol					
amount							
sediment		Methyl Red Test					
Blood Agar:		Urease					
Gelatin Stab:							
Oxygen Requirements:							
Optimum Temperature:							

Student_______________________________

Lab Section_______________________________

Date Started_______________________________

Date Completed_______________________________

Routine Study of Pure Cultures

MORPHOLOGICAL CHARACTERISTICS	DESCRIPTIVE CHART
Cell Shape:	**Organism:**_______________________________
Arrangement:	
Size:	**PHYSIOLOGICAL CHARACTERISTICS**
Spores:	
Gram Stain:	
Motility:	
Capsules:	
Special Stains:	

PHYSIOLOGICAL CHARACTERISTICS

TESTS	RESULTS		
Fermentation:	24 hr	48 hr	72 hr
Glucose			
Lactose			
Sucrose			
Gelatin Liquefaction			

Litmus Milk	Acid	Alk	Coag	red'n	Pept
Reaction:					
Age:					

TESTS	RESULTS
Indole	
Nitrate Reduction	
Hydrogen Sulfide	
Starch Hydrolysis	
Citrate Utilization	
Acetylmethyl Carbinol	
Methyl Red Test	
Urease	

CULTURAL CHARACTERISTICS

Colonies:	
form	
elevation	
surface	
margin	
Agar Slant:	
amount of growth	
form	
consistency	
optical characteristics	
Nutrient Broth:	
surface	
substance	
amount	
sediment	
Blood Agar:	
Gelatin Stab:	
Oxygen Requirements:	
Optimum Temperature:	

Student_______________________________________

Lab Section___________________________________

Date Started__________________________________

Date Completed________________________________

Routine Study of Pure Cultures

MORPHOLOGICAL CHARACTERISTICS		DESCRIPTIVE CHART					
Cell Shape:		Organism:_________________					
Arrangement:		**PHYSIOLOGICAL CHARACTERISTICS**					
Size:							
Spores:		TESTS		RESULTS			
Gram Stain:							
Motility:		Fermentation:		24 hr	48 hr	72 hr	
Capsules:		Glucose					
Special Stains:		Lactose					
		Sucrose					
CULTURAL CHARACTERISTICS		Gelatin Liquefaction					
Colonies:		Litmus Milk	Acid	Alk	Coag	red'n	Pept
form							
elevation							
surface		Reaction:					
margin		Age:					
Agar Slant:		Indole					
amount of growth		Nitrate Reduction					
form							
consistency		Hydrogen Sulfide					
optical characteristics		Starch Hydrolysis					
Nutrient Broth:		Citrate Utilization					
surface							
substance		Acetylmethyl Carbinol					
amount		Methyl Red Test					
sediment							
Blood Agar:		Urease					
Gelatin Stab:							
Oxygen Requirements:							
Optimum Temperature:							

Student_______________________________

Lab Section___________________________

Date Started__________________________

Date Completed________________________

Routine Study of Pure Cultures

MORPHOLOGICAL CHARACTERISTICS	DESCRIPTIVE CHART

Cell Shape:

Arrangement:

Size:

Spores:

Gram Stain:

Motility:

Capsules:

Special Stains:

CULTURAL CHARACTERISTICS

Colonies:
- form
- elevation
- surface
- margin

Agar Slant:
- amount of growth
- form
- consistency
- optical characteristics

Nutrient Broth:
- surface
- substance
- amount
- sediment

Blood Agar:

Gelatin Stab:

Oxygen Requirements:

Optimum Temperature:

Organism:_______________________

PHYSIOLOGICAL CHARACTERISTICS

TESTS	RESULTS		
Fermentation:	24 hr	48 hr	72 hr
Glucose			
Lactose			
Sucrose			
Gelatin Liquefaction			

Litmus Milk	Acid	Alk	Coag	red'n	Pept
Reaction:					
Age:					

Test	Result
Indole	
Nitrate Reduction	
Hydrogen Sulfide	
Starch Hydrolysis	
Citrate Utilization	
Acetylmethyl Carbinol	
Methyl Red Test	
Urease	